MEDICAL JIHAD USA

FEMALE GENITAL MUTILATION

Richard Matteoli

Published by:
Nemean Press
Primo Evinco Te
First Conquer Thyself

Soft Cover ISBN: 978-1-943347-56-8
Hard Cover ISBN: 978-1-943347-57-5

This is a Mandated Report to the Social Body regarding Socialized Violence and Acculturated Child Abuse.

Dedicated to Donna Jean

Images courtesy from Google and Wikipedia.

Acknowledgments: John J. Whitworth

LEGAL CONCEPTS GOVERNING AN INDIVIDUAL'S RIGHTS

Peter S. Stavrianoudakis, Attorney at Law

It must be conceded that a state is not constrained in the exercise of its "police powers" to ignore experience which marks a class of victims nor is it prevented by the "equal protection of the laws" from confirming its restrictions to cases where the need is deemed clearest.

Female Genital Mutilation, as counterpart to circumcision, has laid the gauntlet, by seeking through the proper channels to protect a class of citizens who, to date, have had no voice.

Prescribing a select path for children can be accomplished should the proponents save as limited by constitutional provisions safeguarding individual rights, so that a state may choose means to protect itself and its citizens against criminal or pseudo-criminal violation of its laws and with due regard to the comparative gravity of the criminal offense and whether their consequences are more or less injurious are matters for its determination.

The rational basis equal protection test is not appropriate for the constitutional evaluation of all criminal classification systems.

Within constitutional limits, the legislature with sufficient power to define crime is absolute and command of equal protection leaves no lawmaker much leeway to affect separate groups divergently.

However, should Congressional power wane or exhibit signs of political atrophy, individual States may validly call upon its "police powers" into play and isolate a class of victims, seeking to rectify any perceived wrongs.

THE CALIFORNIA CHILD ABUSE & NEGLECT REPORTING LAW

WHY MUST YOU REPORT?

The primary intent of the reporting law is to protect the child.

WHAT IS CHILD ABUSE?

The Penal Code (P.C.) defines child abuse as "a physical injury which is inflicted by other than accidental means on a child or another person."

(a). A *physical injury* inflicted by other than accidental means on a child. (P.C. 11165.6).

(b). *Willful cruelty or unjustified punishment,* including inflicting or permitting unjustifiable physical pain or mental suffering, or the endangerment of the child's person or health. (P.C. 11165.3). "Mental Suffering" in and of itself is not required to be reported. However, it may be reported. (P.C. 11165.4).

(c). Neglect of a child, whether "severe" or "general," must also be reported if the perpetrator is a person responsible for the child's welfare. It includes acts or omissions harming, or threatening to harm the child's health or welfare. (P.C. 11165.2).

(d). Unlawful corporal punishment or injury, willfully inflicted, resulting in a traumatic condition. (P.C. 11165.4).

WHO REPORTS?

Legally mandated reporters include "child care custodians," "health practitioners," "employees of a child protective agency." And "commercial film and photographic print processors."

State of California
Department of Social Services
Office of Child Abuse Prevention

HIPPOCRATIC OATH[1]

I swear by Apollo the physician, by Aesculapius, and Panacea, and I take to witness all the gods, all the goddesses, to keep according to my abilities and my judgment the following oath.

To consider dear to me as my parents him who taught me this art; to live in common with him and if necessary to share my goods with him; to look upon his children as my own brothers, to teach them this art if they so desire without fee or written promise; to impart to my sons and the sons of the master who taught me and the disciples who have enrolled themselves and have agreed to the rules of the profession, but to these alone, the precepts and the instruction. I will prescribe regimen for the good of my patients according to my ability and my judgment and *never do harm to anyone*. To please no one will I prescribe a deadly drug, nor give, advise which will cause his death. Nor will I give a woman a pessary to procure abortion. But I will preserve the purity of my life and my art. I will not cut for stone, even for patients in whom the disease is manifest; I will leave this operation to be performed by practitioners (specialists in this art). In every house where I come, I will only enter for the good of my patients, keeping myself far from all intentional ill-doing and all seduction, and especially from the pleasures of love with women or men, be they free or slave. All that may come to my knowledge in the exercise of my profession or outside of my profession or in daily commerce with men, which ought not to be spread abroad, I will keep secret and will never reveal. If I keep this oath faithfully, may I enjoy my life and practice my art, respected by all men and in all times; but if I swerve from it or violate it, may the reverse be my lot.

FORWARD

Genital Mutilation is a topic requiring fortitude to concentrate on. It is being forced into non-Islamic countries through a form of Cultural Imperialism. Genital Dismemberments are a form of Incest and must be understood.

We must educate ourselves and others because there is intent to bring this abomination to our daughters. In fact, we must also free our sons from the lie being perpetrated on them from a false acculturation. Even those who practice such things have no knowledge of their origins. Genital Mutilation is a *mock-death* ceremony in *ancestor worship*.

The secret of freedom lies in educating people,
whereas the secret of tyranny is in keeping them ignorant.

Maximilien Robespierre

The child has been fully sexualized before the advent of Freud.

James R. Kincaid

If an injury is to be inflicted on a person,
It is to be so severe, that the person's retaliation, need not be feared.

Niccolo Machiavelli.
The Prince

One of the saddest lessons of history is this: If we've been bamboozled long enough, we tend to reject any evidence of the bamboozle. We're no longer interested in finding out the truth. The bamboozle has captured us. It's simply too painful to acknowledge, even to ourselves, that we've been taken. Once you give a charlatan power over you, you almost never get it back.

Carl Sagan
The Demon-Haunted World: Science as a Candle in the Dark

If I can stop one heart from breaking,
I shall not live in vain;
If I can ease one life from aching,
Or cool one pain,
Or help one fainting robin
Unto his nest again,
I shall not live in vain.

Emily Dickenson

Annabel Lee
Edgar Allen Poe

It was many and many a year ago,
  In a kingdom by the sea,
That a maiden there lived whom you may know
  By the name of Annabel Lee;
And this maiden she lived with no other thought
  Than to love and be loved by me.

I was a child and *she* was a child,
  In this kingdom by the sea,
But we loved with a love that was more than love—
  I and my Annabel Lee—
With a love that the wingèd seraphs of Heaven
  Coveted her and me.

And this was the reason that, long ago,
  In this kingdom by the sea,
A wind blew out of a cloud, chilling
  My beautiful Annabel Lee;
So that her highborn kinsmen came
  And bore her away from me,
To shut her up in a sepulchre
  In this kingdom by the sea.

The angels, not half so happy in Heaven,
   Went envying her and me—
Yes!—that was the reason (as all men know,
   In this kingdom by the sea)
That the wind came out of the cloud by night,
   Chilling and killing my Annabel Lee.

But our love it was stronger by far than the love
   Of those who were older than we—
   Of many far wiser than we—
And neither the angels in Heaven above
   Nor the demons down under the sea
Can ever dissever my soul from the soul
   Of the beautiful Annabel Lee;

For the moon never beams, without bringing me
   dreams
   Of the beautiful Annabel Lee;
And the stars never rise, but I feel the bright eyes
   Of the beautiful Annabel Lee;
And so, all the night-tide, I lie down by the side
   Of my darling—my darling—my life and my bride,
   In her sepulchre there by the sea—
   In her tomb by the sounding sea.

Contents

Introduction

Perhaps the sentiments contained in the following pages
are not yet sufficiently fashionable to procure them general favor.
A long habit of not thinking a thing wrong
gives it a superficial appearance of being right
and raises at first a formidable outcry in defense of custom.
Time makes more converts than reason.

Thomas Paine

Circumcision **in any form** is NOT Islamic, Judaic, nor Christian. It is NOT attributable in any way to United States Native Americans. Yet, Genital Dismemberments have become secular apart from the 3 Abrahamic Religions.

For historic knowledge of Female Genital Mutilation, FGM, one should refer to Dr. Pia Gallo, Padua University, Department of Psychology, Italy.

For an extensive history regarding Genital Dismemberments of both sexes one should reference James DeMeo's texts re: *Sarahasia*.

Comixio Religionis

The mythic tale of Abraham and the fictitious circumcision 'covenant' originated about 550 BCE and spread throughout the Hebrews, eventually infiltrating Islam and then Christianity.[2] All three Jerusalemic religions forbid:

COMIXIO RELIGIONIS: The mixing of religions

The following definitions apply to the religious pitfalls in the three Jerusalemic religions from origination regarding both sexes, both in the meaning of the word circumcision, that is to say: Genital Dismemberments.

This also applies to Humanism's self-deification and the current perversions involving Culture Bound and Culture Specific Syndromes in Gender Reassignment Surgeries.

A phylactery is an amulet with a piece of scripture inside and used in prayer.

BABELIAN IMPERATIVE: **1.** The act of deceiving through use of a euphemism. **2.** The use of language in deception through obfuscation

PHYLACTRY FALSE: false and/or improper use of scripture

Personal Relationship with the Deity

Edward Edinger wrote:[3]

The Self is the ordering and unifying center of the total psyche (Conscious and Unconscious) just as the ego is the center of the conscious personality. Or, put in other words, the ego is the seat of the *subjective* identity while the Self is the seat of the *objective* identity. The Self is the supreme psychic authority and subordinates the ego to it. The Self is most simply described as the inner empirical deity and is identical with the *imago Dei*. ...

Since there are two autonomous centers of psychic being, the relation between the two centers becomes vitally important, ...

Indeed, the myth can be seen as a symbolic expression of the ego-Self relationship.

I, Made God, Make Me Do It

Ancestor Worship – (Veneration)

Ancestor worship is also referred to as ancestor veneration. It is the ritual practice that shows respect to departed family members and dedication to them.

These customs are deeply entrenched worldwide. Different forms range from ceremonies, feasts and sacred monuments. Daily offerings are included.

Many world cultures it has been pivotal in religious practice. Mainly the belief there is a powerful kinship of forefathers and those living in the present. This promotes and strengthens family continuity and transcending morality.

It has been found to have been practiced since the Neolithic Period.[4] Motivations include: respect and love for the dead; fear of the spirits of the dead; and, belief in the continued existence and power of the ancestors to influence the living.

Ancestor worship varies and adapts to their cultural environments.[5] It is still practiced in various forms throughout the world. In many Asian cultures there are annual festivals that honor the dead. Ancestral altars are common.[6]

This practice highly impacts social structure and their norms of the society. It reinforces familial hierarchies and generational respect.[7] The thought of ancestor presence with their authority gives a moral compass that guides descendant behavior. It also combines with and influences religious practices and beliefs.

Syncretism occurs when ancestor veneration often coexists with and enhances other religious practices. This can lead to afterlife beliefs that reflects cultural views of death.

Social and non-religious functions of ancestor veneration help cultivate kinship vales, filial piety, family loyalty, and continuity of family lineage as to be a Jew one's mother must be a Jew.

In this, genital blood rituals are feminine based in menstrual symbolism with fertility overtones. The feminine is dominate in this team predation while the males who advocate are recessive component to maintain the social order for her. They constitute Partial Human Sacrifice in a mock-death ritual commonly called circumcision.

Carl Jung stated of the mother-bond relationship in his study on sacrifice that:[8]

> The libido which builds up religious structures regress in the last analysis to the mother, and thus represents the real bond through which we are connected to its origins. ...
>
> The hero when dead is back in the mother.

Spirituality is, Theology explains, Religion practices

False Native American Excuse

95:4 Surah At-Tin (The Fig): Certainly, _We_ created man in the best make.

Female Genital Mutilations are being introduced into the United States through Islam, and attempting to use Native American Non-Genital rituals as equivalency.

The Native American _Ghost Dance_ and their _Vow to the Sun_ ceremony along with Middle Eastern Genital Blood Rituals, concerning _Circumcision_, will illustrate differences in each, that affect legality. Genital Blood Ritual Dismemberments are a form of Munchausen Syndrome a Factitious Disorder in ancestor worship as mock-death incest.

This last third category and its effects on the American Judicial system through a Medical Jihad are disconcerting by the Judicial acceptance and promulgation of Child Abuse and Molestation. All three are steeped in Conditions as Shared Psychotic Behavior with Delusional Disorder.[9],[10]

Recognized tribes have Separate Nation Status.

Ghost Dance

The Ghost Dance tradition began in the late 1860's by the Western Paiute Indians. It is a male dance signifying a regeneration of the spirits and the beginning of a new earth. The male dances by _himself with no interference_ yet was performed in front of others in the group.

Being regenerative puts the ceremony in the Wise Woman's anima's Life/Death/Life cycle.[11] People act in Servancy, willful duty, to the maternal tribal blood/flesh unit.

The *Ghost Dance* initially considered living in faith, an honest life, peaceful adjustments with the whites all within the natural superiority of the Indians.

Dancers would be transported to the afterworld where departed ancestors resided living in the pre-reservation old happy days with abundant bison.[12],[13],[14] The Ghost Dance involves the standard Native circular movement. Circles are signs of matriarchal influence.

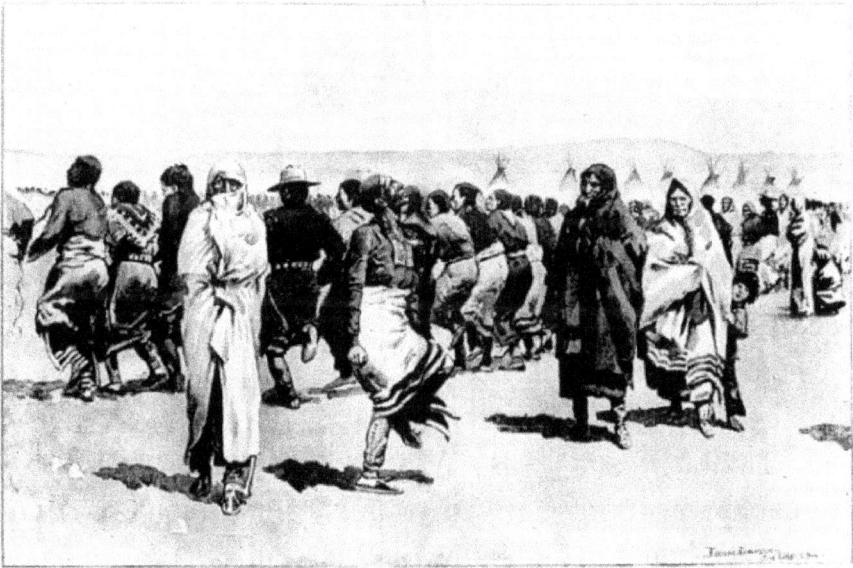

Ghost Dance, Ogallala Sioux, Pine Ridge, 1890.

Later for some in conflict with the white men, as Wounded Knee, those who performed the Ghost Dance believed they were making themselves immune from the white man's bullets.

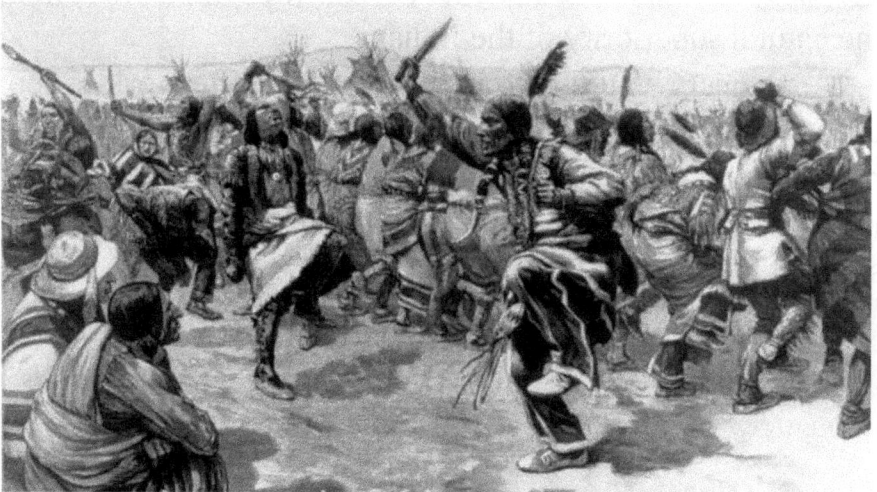

Sioux at Wounded Knee, London News, engraving 1891.
Library of Congress.

The Dance was initiated by a dreamer Wodziwob who died in 1872 and the Ghost Dance slowly lost favor for some. The blood aspect that came later was from a son of Wodziwob's assistant Tavibo.

Tavibo's son was Wovoka and he self-inflicted Stigmata to his body derived from Mormon theology. This encouraged belief in him being the Messiah as a type of Christ figure who has come to the Native Americans.

The massacre at Wounded Knee brought outrage in the eastern part of the United States. Public dissent caused a reestablishment of many broken Treaties with the benefits.

The Bureau of Indian Affairs banned the Ghost Dance though it continued in various degrees, much of which was underground – not public to outsiders.

With social changes the second Ghost Dance continues for some, but much of the harshness and bloodletting has ceased. The Navajo considered it worthless words.

Sun Dance

Origins of the Sun Dance is unclear and possibly Centuries old. It involves group worship with *males only making the sacrificial blood ritual as well as preparing celebrant males* by placing hooks in the flesh and threading sinews through the body as between the tendons. The ceremony was Illustrated in both *A Man Called Horse* films.[15]

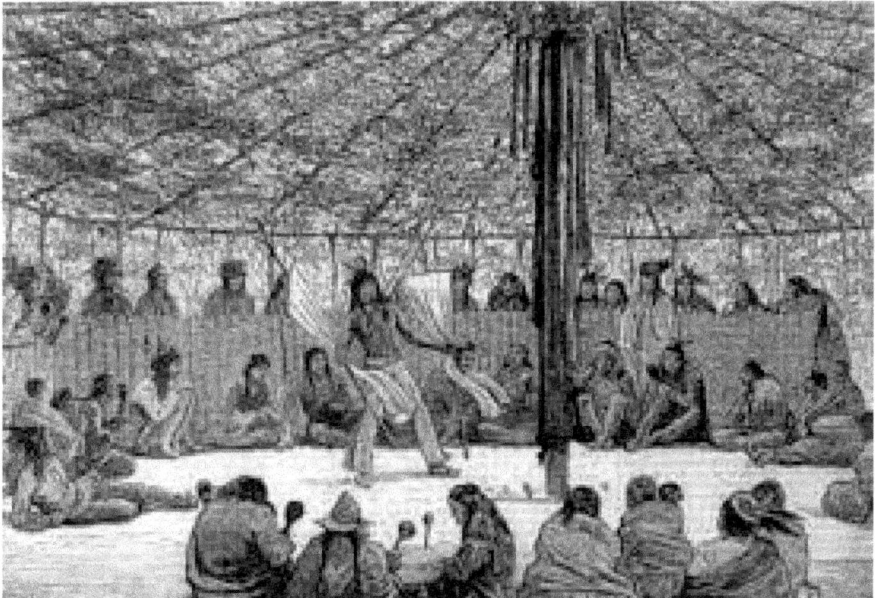

NOTE two diagonal lines that are ropes with hooks attached to the standing man's chest.

The Sun Dance represents both personal and community sacrifice reaffirming the universal and supernatural. The ritual was augmented with prayers and offerings that reflected secular and religious aspirations.

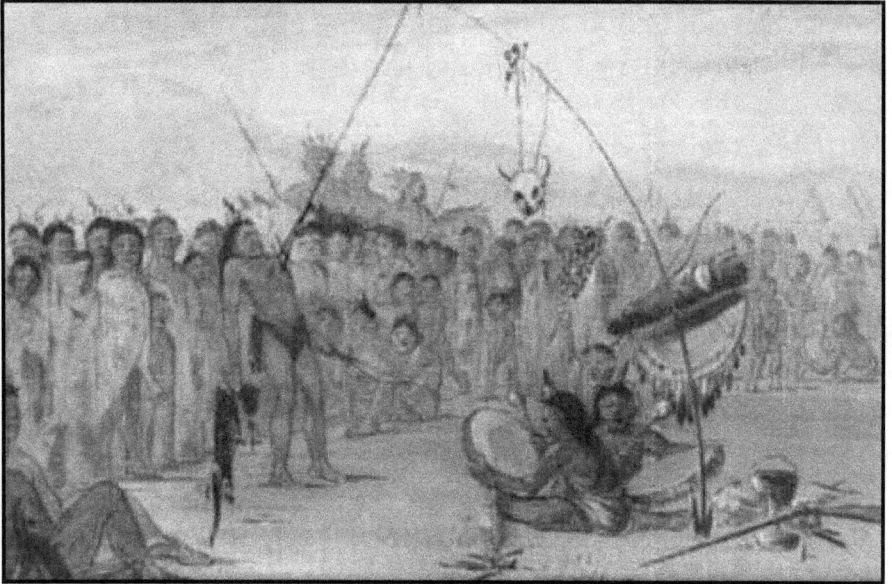

Britannica 1841

Before the Battle of Little Big Horn, Sioux chief Sitting Bull performed a Sun Dance with the aid of his brother cutting 50 pieces of flesh from each arm. He danced until he passed out. Upon awakening he related his vision that the Native people would defeat General Custer.

Joseph Campbell in *The Power of Myth* stated the Sun Dance participant's chant was:

We must suffer as woman suffers.[16]

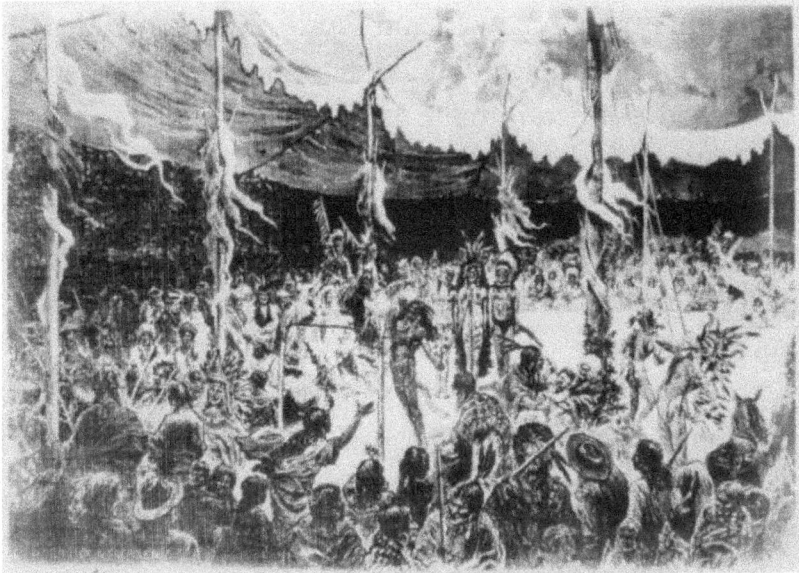

Sioux 1874. Multiple participants.

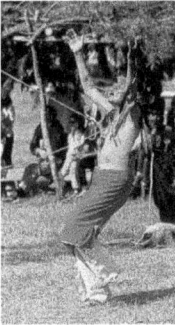

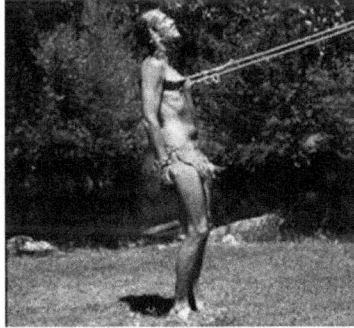

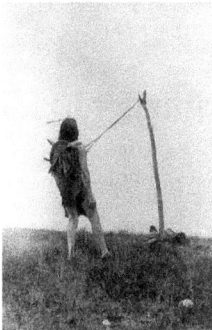

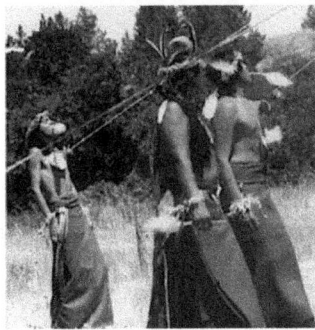

Sacred pain, renewal, and sacrifice are ritual themes in rites like the Sun Dance. Blood is an important element and must be incorporated into the Sun Dance ritual.

Outside Native America, so too, any-and-all ritual genital dismemberments, whether total or partial. Worldwide social forms of blood rituals, however performed, reside heavily in menstrual symbolism along with being Flesh and Blood ceremonies.

Mythically speaking the Flesh and the Blood belong to the individual as well as the group's Anima identity. The feminine anima and masculine animus both reside within every individual. Currently, many tribes request non-Native individuals not to attend their renewed ritual.

In 1978 President Jimmy Carter signed the *American Indian Religious Freedom Act (1978)*. Both the Ghost Dance and the Vow to the Sun are legally protected under the First Amendment along with Freedom of Religion.

Yet the excision of flesh and blood letting has greatly subsided, though still required, to being somewhat non-existent in comparison to the times performed during the United States expansion into taking sovereignty over their lands.

Detroit Jihad: Judge Bernard Friedman on Female Genital Mutilation

The Feminine Determines the Social Genitals

Judge Bernard Friedman ruled Female Genital Mutilation of children has the same rights as the ***adult male only*** Native American Ghost Dance and Vow to the Sun rituals without taking into consideration today's limited nature of the ceremonies.

Judge Friedman basically appears to be a consenting Child Molesting pimp for his own misguided religious butchery. Or, just plain ignorant.

He did so to protect his Jewish faith's Genital Dismemberment of male circumcision, which is actually Pre-Dynastic Egyptian.

If Judge Friedman did not follow his religious dictates by associating the Native American male only rituals he would have been ostracized from the Jewish community.

Female Genital Dismemberment originated in the African areas of Somalia and Kenya prior to Dynastic Egypt.

The main court Drs. in the Detroit case was Dr. Jumana Nagarwala and her associate Dr. Fakhruddin Attah.

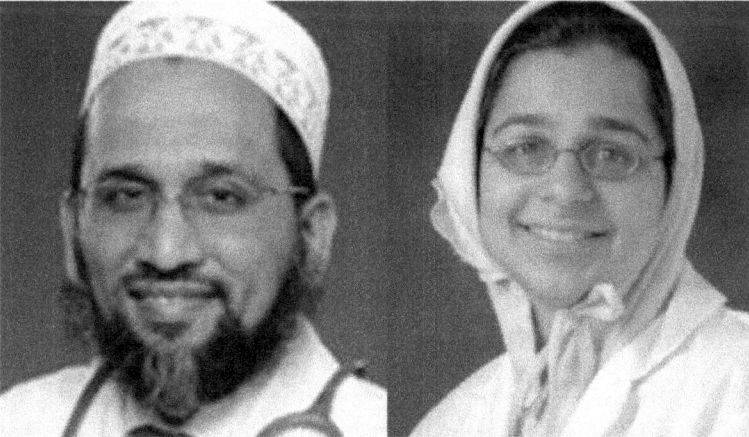

Dr. Fakhruddin Attah - Dr. Jumana Nagarwala.

American Medical Jihad

Ultimately, the Child Judges the Parent.

Bringing Female Genital Mutilation into the United States is projecting power relations that Islam terms *Hijra*.[17],[18],[19] *Hijra* in the Indian subcontinent is a generic term including **<u>genetically transexual women with Congenital Adrenal Hyperplasia</u>**. It forces acceptance by associating its validity to Jewish male only circumcision and Native American male only rituals and not Jerusalemic.[20]

USA's male circumcision motif was through medicalization from perversions and improper medical studies of Judaism, yet first onto Islam in the 15th Century, then now with Christianity finalized in the mid-20th century.

Dismemberments of both sexes in genital blood rituals, is socialized violence and abusive behavior that has irrationally gained a foothold of the populations collective psyche.[21] Further, these Dismemberments involve a Societal type of Stockholm Syndrome.

Psychologically they are used as tension relieving forms of entertainment through Thanatos. Thanatos, sometimes called a Death Wish, is the motif used. Thanatos is normal and much stronger than the Pleasure Principal related to the survival instinct.

Genital rituals reside in the psychopathy of the Munchausen Complex, a Factitious Disorder. Ritualistically it occurs with the minor being separated into a prescribed ritual space by adults where the amputations occur.

Rarely does the ritual occur by the individual alone. The Munchausen Complex involves, in part the following behaviors: Social Transference, Transgenerational, Collective Transmission, Social Agency and for Profit.

Circumcision performed on a person under legal age of consent is child abuse and molestation with an Intent to Disfigure. Circumcision is a socially validated form of entertainment used and justified in psychological conditions and pathologic behavior. Genital rituals are developed so that anyone may participate using their own particular quirk.

Being a body marking, the dismembered sexual organ becomes a tribal marking forever, fixating the victim to the social group and identity. As such, abuse is then generationally passed down. The Totem Penis and Totem Vulva are carved in flesh instead of wood.

Also, it feeds personal and social collective narcissism which in turn leads to an altering of both, again individual and social morality, moral tribalism, via obtuse justifications.[22],[23]

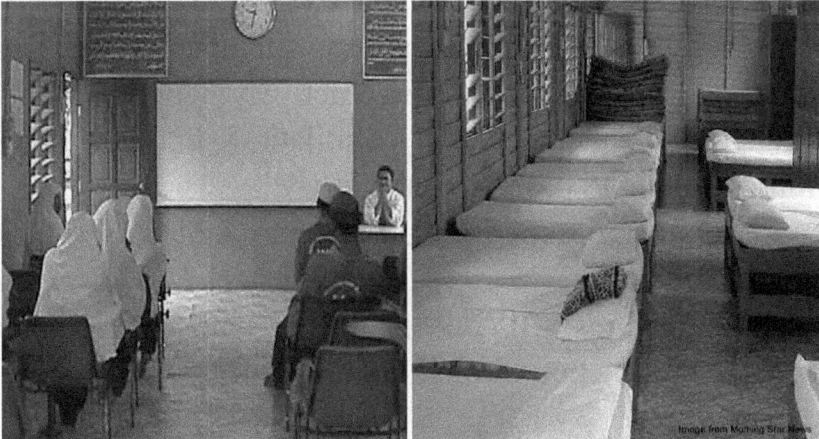

Forced Pakistani Female Islamic Religious Rehabilitation Center

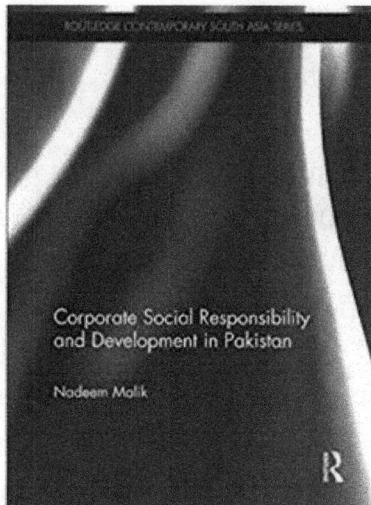

Corporate Social Responsibility
and Development in Pakistan

Nadeem Malik

Required Corporate-Social Practices According to Islam

Sacramento, California

A combined example of Ethical Drift, Ethical Fading and Moral Disengagement using Parallel Construction (see: Conditions), with multiple motifs, is well illustrated by the Catholic nun's Sisters of Mercy hospital; Dignity Health in Sacramento.

A group of Muslim physicians attempted to Censure a veteran patient they knew was actively working against introducing Female Genital Mutilation into the USA. Families belong to professional clans.

Sacramento Superior Court supports them by refusing to review evidence. Mercy Hospital group, *Dignity Health*, including facilities affiliated in unison with each other all worked to silence him through punishment.

Dignity Health was fined $37 Million by both California and Federal Departments of Justice for falsifying claims regarding x-military Tricare insurance patients with heart disease and sending them to psychiatry.[24]

When that one veteran cardiac patient strenuously objected, he lost his 2nd Amendment Rights in Superior Court.

Dr. Sultan Ahmad Sultan lost his Dignity Health hospital privileges after over drugging a patient and sending him to psychiatry. Dr. Sherwin Valadkhani of the Ayatollah Khomeini medical school pledged to practice under Islamic precepts whose first name was Mohammad and changed it to Sherwin after four rape and assault charges in Texas. Dr. Amer Ali of Baqui University in Pakistan lied in his statements. Dr. Saddiqi whose name have many variants belongs to another clan of Pakistani doctors. Dr. Ramy Ramsis Girgis is a Southern California transexual who gives psychiatric evaluations to support the Dignity Health Islamic group without patient contact. Dr. Janek Mehtani has been found to have routinely overprescribed medicines. Dr. M. JBS Behniwal has been convicted of exposing himself to a patient and had her masturbate him in his office. Licensed nurse Mohammad Kamal Merbaa with non-Muslim Drs. Rachael Smith and Maria Lewis and Physician Assistant Cheyenne Booth and licensed Clinical Social Workers Cheryl Marie Camarena and Amy C. White aided.

Regarding the patient, the day before he took out his dining room carpet, cut it down to put in his pick-up truck and then went to the dumps. Returning home he then laid cement in his back yard. The next day he had a cardiology appointment and they sent him to the hospital for low blood pressure. He was a dehydrated veteran with a pacemaker.

At the hospital besides saline, he was given the following meds: chlorpromazine, haloperidol (haldol), hydralazine, hydrocodone, naloxone, morphine, olanzapine (risperidone), ondansetron, and prochloperazine and then sent to psych.

Later in psych he was given the following meds: benzotropine, bisacodyl, benxotropine, chlorpromazine, diocusate, glanzapine, hydroxyzine, lorazepam, morphine, naloxone, olanzaprine, ondansetaon, prochlorperazine, visteral, zofran, and zyprexa.

All this for a case of dehydration. *He had no chance.*

Also, Dignity Health has an in-house Continuing Education course on Female Genital Mutilation. This gives credits required toward maintaining State licensure. Considering their history, it is advised to make it Mandatory to maintain employment.

Other Catholic nuns in England also circumcised as a habit before those in the USA. One motif challenged may use another motif as a form of retaliation and Defensive Functioning to avoid the consequences of improper behavior with improper diagnoses including Telehealth.

QU'RAN

Herve Bertaux-Navoiseau found in the *Qu'ran* verses to argue against Islamic mutilations:[25]

3: 6 It is He who forms you in the wombs however He wills. There is no deity except Him, the Exalted in Might, the Wise.

3: 191b "Our Lord, You did not create this aimlessly;

4: 118-119 They call upon instead of Him none but **female [deities]**, and they [actually] call upon none but a rebellious Satan. Whom Allah has cursed. For he had said, "I will surely take from among Your servants a specific portion. And I will mislead them, and I will arouse in them [sinful] desires, and I will command them so they will slit the ears of cattle, and I will command them so they will change the creation of Allah."

10: 59 b Say, "Has Allah permitted you [to do so], or do you invent [something] about Allah?

16: 116 And do not say about what your tongues assert of untruth. "This is lawful and this is unlawful," to invent falsehood about Allah. Indeed, those who invent falsehood about Allah will not succeed.

25: 2 To Whom belongs the Kingdom of the heavens and the earth, and He has not taken Him a child, and He has no associate in the Kingdom; and He created everything, so He has determined it in (exact) measure.

27: 88 Now you see the mountains, thinking they are firmly fixed, but they are travelling ʹjustʹ like clouds. ʹThat isʹ the design of Allah, Who has perfected everything. Surely He is All-Aware of what you do.

30: 30b No change should there be in the creation of Allah. That is the correct religion, but most of the people do not know.

32: 7-9 Who has perfected everything He created. And He originated the creation of humankind from clay.[1] Then He made his descendants from an extract of a humble fluid, then He fashioned them and had a spirit of His Own ˹creation˺ breathed into them. And He gave you hearing, sight, and intellect. ˹Yet˺ you hardly give any thanks.

40: 61 It is Allāh who made for you the night that you may rest therein and the day giving sight. Indeed, Allāh is full of bounty to the people, but most of the people are not grateful.

64: 3 He created the heavens and the earth for a purpose. He shaped you ˹in the womb˺, perfecting your form. And to Him is the final return.

82: 6 O man! What has deceived you about your generous Lord.

Islam's crux is that they are a masculine religion. They are as a step-father to wife Judaism and son Christianity. The first father YHWY with the advent of Christ in the mythic tradition of Osiris and other mythic paternal figures who have become dispossessed are castrates.

Islam believes that the moon is masculine and the sun is feminine. This is backward and possibly derived from envy and jealousy of the feminine experience. Gyno-resentment leads to active misogyny with masculine glorifications.

Prior to activation of the male dismemberments, he lived in societies that possessed Andro-resentment which, in the male genital dismemberments represent active misandry with feminine menstrual glorifications.

The feminine self's Gyno-resentment was made out of jealousy by non-African women who migrated south during the drying of the Sahara whose genitals were not as pronounced as the African women's genitals. Female Genital Mutilations were not from masculine misogyny. They were more likely than not initiated on female African slaves living in the households of the Holy Land immigrants around the time of the Saharan drying.

According to Islam the moon is masculine and superior and stronger than the feminine sun. By trying to take the power of the moon upon, and within, himself he becomes frustrated himself and all those around him. Judaism's Toiletry=Menstrual-Hut is Israel. A place not for true men and unprotected children.

And yet Islam still enslaves and castrate black African males as well as non-believers. Islam also is allowed to rape little girls according to Jewish female deity precepts.

The urge to save humanity is almost always only
a false-face for the urge to rule it.
H. L. Mencken

Ethics

**Rituals are adult games that should not be
forced upon children**

ETHICAL DRIFT, FADING, MORAL DISENGAGEMENT

Ethical Drift and *Ethical Fading* are incremental deviations from ethical practice that goes unnoticed by individuals who justify the deviations as acceptable and who believe themselves to be maintaining their ethical boundaries.[26],[27]

Ethical Drift and *Ethical Fading* escalate imperceptibly until even major breaches are rationalized as reasonable. Four intrusions may be:

1) where there is intense competition.
2) with competition other members of the group may encourage the violator to continue.
3) people feel they are in a zero-sum game.
4) people see no way out of the quandary.

Ethical Drift may be quick as with a new, though false, medical treatment including even vaccines.

Ethical Fading often occurs insidiously without conscious awareness. Environmental forces predominately provoke. We rarely mean to do the wrong thing, but subtle cues lead us to ignore the moral implications of our decisions. *Ethical Fading* is one of the reasons there is a gap between how we intend to act and how we actually end up behaving. *We let our ethics fade from view.*[28]

Moral Disengagement leads to values and standards being altered. Assault and Battery of the genitals of those who are of minor age is such a case.[29]

Eight dimensions of Moral Disengagement are:

1) moral justification
2) euphemistic labelling
3) advantageous comparison
4) displacement of responsibility
5) diffusion of responsibility
6) distortion of consequences
7) dehumanization
8) attribution of blame

People usually do not ask themselves if they are acting unethically. They will resort to rationalizations as "It is God's will," "I was forced to do it," or "They deserved it," or "I did it for their own good." As well as, "It was strictly business," or "I did it for the safety of the organization."

ETHICAL DRIFT: Ethical Drift involves an incremental deviation from ethical practice that goes unnoticed by individuals who justify the deviations as acceptable and who believe themselves to be maintaining their ethical boundaries.

ETHICAL FADING: Ethical Fading is a form of self-deception. It occurs when we subconsciously avoid or disguise the moral implications of a decision. It allows us to behave in immoral ways while maintaining the conviction that we are good, moral people.

MORAL DISENGAGEMENT: Moral Disengagement refers to the process where an individual or group of people distances themselves from the normal or usual ethical standards of behavior and then become convinced that new unethical behaviors are justified often due to some perceived extenuating circumstances.

ETHICS: **1.** Moral principles that govern a person's behavior or the conducting of an activity. **2.** The branch of knowledge that deals with moral principles.

MORAL: of or relating to principles of right and wrong in behavior: ethical expressing or teaching a conception of right behavior.

ALTRUISTIC ETHOS: a postulated form of argument or discussion to enhance a belief or position as it relates to humanity in general

SELECTIVE ETHOS: a postulated form of argument or discussion to enhance a belief or position that usually separates one person or group of persons from another person or group of persons usually via perceived innate differences between them, and often contains deceptions from altruistic posturing with subsequent actions in Situation Ethics, which is a Fallacy.

SITUATIONAL ETHICS: the doctrine of flexibility in the application of moral laws according to circumstances.

SUPERNATURALISM: a belief in an otherworldly realm or reality that, in one way or another, is commonly associated with all forms of religion.

SUBJECTIVISM: Subjectivism in ethics suggests that moral statements are only ever the opinion and experience of the person saying the statement, and collective moral opinions come about when many people agree on ethical matters.

CONSEQUENTIALISM: Consequentialism is an ethical theory that judges whether or not something is right by what its consequences are.

INTUITIONALISM: Institutional ethics (a.k.a. organizational ethics) refers to the application of ethics in such institutions as hospitals, professional organization, and corporations. It regards institutions as moral agents with responsibilities and accountability.

EMOTIVISM: the view that moral judgments do not function as statements of fact but rather as expressions of the speaker's or writer's feelings.

DUTY-BASED ETHICS: Duty-based ethics teaches that some acts are right or wrong because of the sorts of things they are, and people have a duty to act accordingly, regardless of the good or bad consequences that may be produced.

VIRTUE ETHICS: Virtue ethics is an approach that treats virtue and character as the primary subjects of ethics, in contrast to other ethical systems that put consequences of voluntary acts, principles or rules of conduct, or obedience to divine authority in the primary role.

SITUATION ETHICS: In Situation Ethics right and wrong depend on the situation. There are no universal moral rules or rights. Each case is unique and deserves a unique solution. Situation Ethics rejects prefabricated decisions and prescriptive rules.

NORMATIVE (PRESCRIPTIVE) ETHICS: Normative Ethics is the study of ethical behavior that investigates questions regarding how one ought to act, in a moral sense. It asks: How should people act?

APPLIED ETHICS: Applied Ethics (a.k.a. Practical Ethics) is the application of ethics to real-world problems, attempting to answer the question of how people should act in specific situations. It asks: How do we take moral knowledge and put it into practice?

META-ETHICS: The study of the meanings of ethical terms, the nature of ethical judgments, and the types of ethical argument. It asks: What does 'right' even mean?

DESCRIPTIVE ETHICS: Descriptive Ethics (a.k.a. comparative ethics) is the study of people's beliefs about morality. It asks: What do people think is right?

DISPLACEMENT OF RESPONSIBILITY: Displacement of responsibility is when people avoid feeling responsibility for unethical behavior by shifting responsibility for those actions on others.

DEHUMANIZATION: is the process of depriving a person or group of positive human qualities

DIFFUSION OF RESPONSIBILITY: Diffusion of Responsibility is a sociopsychological phenomenon where a person is less likely to take responsibility for action or inaction when other bystanders or witnesses are present. Considered a form of attribution where the individual assumes that others either are responsible for taking action or have already done so.

Diffusion of responsibility refers to the decreased responsibility of each member of the group feels when they are part of a group.

Assumption of responsibility tends to decrease when the potential helping group is larger, resulting in little aiding behavior by the bystanders. Put in other words, this is the fact that as the number of bystanders increases, the personal responsibility that an individual bystander decreases, thus so does his or her tendency to help decreases.

Ethics is the difference between what you have a right to do and what is right to do.
Potter Stewart.

A man without ethics is a wild beast loosed upon this world.
Albert Camus

Conditions

The Child has a right to retaliate

Parallel Construction – legal

Parallel Construction is a subterfuge operation used by law enforcement in building a parallel, separate, criminal investigation in order to conceal how and why an investigation began. Evidence laundering, concealing evidence, is when one officer obtains evidence in violation of the 4th Amendment then passes it to another officer who gets it accepted in court. Laundering includes falsifications.[30]

Illegally obtained evidence is inadmissible in court due to the doctrine of Fruit of the Poisonous Tree. Further falsified conclusions passed down to others who depend on truthful investigations are then easily used as facts and more blame is exacerbated upon an innocent individual. In Medicine this is inclusive to Misdiagnosis and innocent prosecution of a patient the doctors do not agree with though the patient may have called medical misbehavior. Was further illustrated in Sacramento section of previous Islam chapter.

Psychological Projection

Psychological Projection is an *ego defensive mechanism* in denying impulses and attributing them to others. It is accusing others what the person themselves are doing. Similarly, this includes such behaviors as Blame Shifting. What the ego repudiates is split from the Self and then put on another. That other person may be the person who brought forth their improper behavior as a means of retaliation and an attempt to maintain innocence and be free themselves of prosecution.[31],[32]

This has occurred in Sacramento California at Mercy Hospital by a physician, in part, who went to the Iranian Ayatollah Khomeini medical school whose vowed educational precept is to practice and expand medicine according to Islamic religious practices.

Machiavellianism

Machiavellianism in the realm of personality psychology, not the political philosophy of the same name, is a trait revolving on manipulation, callousness and an indifference to morality. As such there is no Cognitive Dissonance. In Islam it is within their religious proscription to lie and deceive non-believers because doing so is not a sin but honored. This is termed *Taqiyya*.

Motivation exhibits cold detachment, selfishness, using others as objects to be used as tools to enhance oneself and/or the Self's identified Group through low emotional intelligence and lack of empathy. Machiavellianism, narcissism (in part genetic) and psychopathy make up what some psychologists term the Dark Triad.[33]

Gaslighting

Gaslighting is a form of abuse. Similar to Machiavellianism it manipulates. Here a person plants seeds of doubts in an individual or a target group. The objective is to affect memories, perceptions, one's own sanity, in persistent denial, misdirection, contradictions and lying. The purpose is to destabilize, disorient and delegitimize the victim as well as their belief systems.

Gaslighting is particularly observable in psychiatry and their institutions. Denial of previous abuses to staging of bizarre events is common Defensive Functioning.[34],[35]

Disorienting the victim also includes those around the victim and the organization(s) including all things medical within the context of a medical Jihad.

A victim's ability to resist manipulations relies on the victim trusting their own judgment. Yet the victim's ability to defend themselves is minimal.[36]

Fear Conditioning

Pavlovian fear conditioning is a behavioral paradigm in which organisms learn to predict aversive events.[37]

Fear Conditioning maintains an abusive social order. It is a form of learning in which an aversive stimulus (e.g. an electrical shock) is associated with a particular neutral context (e.g., a room) or neutral stimulus (e.g., a tone), resulting in the expression of fear responses to the originally neutral stimulus or context.

This can be done by pairing the neutral stimulus with an aversive stimulus (e.g., an electric shock, loud noise, or unpleasant odor).[38] Eventually, the neutral stimulus alone can elicit the state of fear.

In the vocabulary of classical conditioning, the neutral stimulus or context is the "conditional stimulus" (CS), the aversive stimulus is the "unconditional stimulus" (US), and the fear is the "conditional response" (CR). Fear.

Conditioned fear can be inherited. Research has shown that neuroanatomical changes to the body have been proven to be inherited from parents.

Bullying

Bullying uses force actual to implied. With success organized Fear Conditioning is instilled. The behavior is often repeated and becomes habitual. The more it is used, habituation may rest in an established dominating social order within the projection of authority. Bullying employs force, coercion, threats and intimidation.

Motivations of bullies and their accomplices may be from envies and resentments from issues in self-esteem to conceal shame or anxiety from an inflated yet fragile ego.

Peer Groups often encourage bullying while themselves engage in behaviors as mocking, excluding, hitting and insulting as sources of entertainment. With in-group use toward those perceived to them as outsiders Group Codependence develops in the group. Bullying is often seen unabated in abusive societies.

Through Moral Tribalism Denial of Due Process with Suborning Justice, the angst of Cognitive Dissonance is greatly reduced. Collective Bullying, also termed a Bullying Culture and Mobbing, can arise in any context where people come together whether in school, workplace, home, neighborhoods, familial, social, or to the national.

From verbal harassment to physical assault the Scapegoat's onus is rationalized within the Scapegoat's identity be it: race, religion, gender, sexual orientation, social class, appearance, behavior, personality, reputation, lineage, size, strength, ability and/or body language.

Adults who bully often possess an authoritarian, and punitive, personality synergized with a need to control and dominate.

Bystanders who are best able to inhibit bullying are members of a Support Group. If not stopped a Culture of Bullying will develop and behavior will become the norm. Same with circumcision from whatever motifs it is introduced.[39],[40],[41]

Child Sexual Abuse Accommodation Syndrome, (CSAAS)

Sadly, CSAAS refers to a myriad of symptoms and behavior patterns exhibited by victims of sexual abuse. Victim behaviors, accommodating their abuse, are five in general.[42]

First, secrecy so that the offense does not become known - censorship.

Second, the victim is helpless and whatever they do would be futile.

Third, the victim feels they are trapped - entrapment. This is where the victim accommodates the crimes being committed against them because it has been made futile to resist.

Fourth, often delayed, reaction is disclosure though the disclosure appears conflicted and unconvincing.

Fifth, is retraction of the disclosure.

Transfer of Aggression within Displacement (psychology)

Displaced Aggression appears to be an in-born emotion and is an aggression on other people who are ignorant and unaware of the situation that caused the annoyance.

According to Amina Alhassan, often when women become annoyed at their husbands, they transfer their aggression onto the children.

This is a possible truth with circumcision when Abraham had a son with his concubine.

This is most definitely the entire theme of the Heracles saga from conception to death. Male dismemberment myths are all historically from a goddess.[43]

Cultural Imperialism

Cultural Imperialism is the imposition by one usually politically, economically and/or religious community onto another. It's cultural in that their religion, traditions social and moral norms as well as other aspects are distinct from the systems of the invaded social order. Often Cultural Imperialism used military force yet military force has lost to better forms through many other means

In Islam it is *Hijra* in bringing Female Genital Mutilation to the West, not just the United States of America alone. The current Hijra was preceded and still maintained by false Jewish medical studies.[44] Islam historically conquers through immigration.

The process appears simple, but there are many facets required with various forms of intensity. Conditions to consider, in part are: Cultural Appropriation, Group Dynamics, Peer Pressure, Groupthink, Communal Behavior, Structuration, Social Norm, Mores and Meme Bonding.

Also, in Social Psychology there are factors as: Association, Social Order, possible Comixio Religionis, Object Person, little Reflected Self-Image, Social Justification, Dependency, and Assertions.

Object Person

An *object person* is someone who has been dehumanized due to an attribute or physical quality they possess. Body modifications or sacrifices, for the most part, are accepted by the Object Person if those social practices do not alter what the parson sees as their social purpose.

If the Object Person objects, then psychological inner conflict occurs. The perpetrator is the ritual agent. This inhibits the original social act and the perpetrator must then resort to making claims and arguments in support of their *Social Ideal* as a counter *moral force* to inhibit the object person's moral prostrations. Or the perpetrating *Social Force* may impose repression.

Repression creates opposing Social Values that must eventually be resolved. *Moral Standards* are a part of social values that are often upheld by manipulative arguments that do not allow comment. The *Social Purpose* is maintained.

Making the genitals the Social Object targets the most private, intimate, sensual, and vulnerable part of the body. In this, the child, or adult person is objectified at that moment in time and space in the eyes of the Social Body.[45]

Dependency

Dependency is often the tendency of an individual or individuals to rely on others for advice, guidance, or support. It also is being abnormally tolerant to and dependent on something that is psychologically or physically habit-forming (especially alcohol or narcotic drugs).

Dependency indicates that people can be opportunists: they can be used personally and socially, for another's selfish gratification and fulfillment.

This leads to *conflict* when needs, wants, desires, and perceptions among individuals and socially or groups differ. It drives people, both individually and socially, to *impose* their conceptual way of life onto the dependent persons.

Reasons and excuses to perpetrate abuse are easy to justify through moral doctrines and codes such as commandments and covenants. When successful, social movements overwhelm individual choice, free will, and human rights.

Interdependence

Interdependence is dependence of two or more people or other things on each other. This indicates a higher form of socialization.

Interdependence entails personal and societal responsibilities. We subsist through monetary reward and occupations that are more than simple jobs; they carry significant responsibilities.

Ideally, medicine and religion are businesses that we would prefer to be service-oriented rather than selfish. Medical personnel and religious representatives would hopefully serve the community.

The question we must always ask is whether the occupation's "service" or contribution to society is more beneficial, mischievous, or harmful.

Assertions

To be an acceptable member of a group, a person needs to conform to codes of conduct (cohort codes) that make them acceptable. In this, the social organization adopts official positions.

Genital Dismemberment of healthy infant genital tissue is erroneously justified through the manipulative self-justificatory advice of self-proclaimed medical authority figures.

The advice to circumcise, a form of Genital Dismemberment, comes from selfish impulses. For the female it is worse when beyond the cliteroidectomy. The pharaonic female circumcision will give a lifetime of menstrual and pelvic pain, and up to 20 minutes to urinate.

Reportable complication rate is only documented at the time of surgery until the patient leaves the operation room. After leaving the operation room anything is NOT a reportable event.

For males there is at least a 9%-10% meatal stenosis rate that occurs only to circumcised boys and the figure rises to a minimum 14% complication rate – far higher than any benefit claimed for the surgery. [46]

Constructive Displacement

According to Dr. Janet Menage of the United Kingdom Constructive Displacement is the psychological ability to take a scalpel and cut a patient for their own good and other procedures when pain has a high degree of certainty.

Displacement

Displacement is the transfer of negative feelings from one person or thing to another. Displacement is when a person deals with the tension or anxiety associated with negative feelings, such as fear or anger, by releasing them on a nonthreatening target, → as the genitals of a child.

Behaviors that can be associated with Displacement, in part, include:

Avoidance dismisses uncomfortable thoughts or feelings by staying away from people, places or situations associated with them.

Denial occurs when continuing to engage in behaviors that may be damaging while dismissing the real-life consequences of the action or situation.

Humor is used by reducing, resisting, or hiding negative emotions that may result from a situation by joking about the subject.

Projection, again, is attributing a person's behavior and shortcomings to someone else.

Regression occurs when a person returns to behaviors from an earlier stage of life.

Rationalization is justifying behavior by attempting to provide a rational explanation.

Doubling

Dr. Robert Lifton wrote *The Nazi Doctors* introducing the term Doubling for the psychological split that allowed them to commit atrocities while still behaving normally at home.[47]

If you are curing a sickness anything is possible. The image of cure lends itself to the restorative myth of state violence and to the literal enactment of the myth... The key to understanding how Nazi doctors came to do the work of Auschwitz is the psychological principle I call **doubling**: the division of the self into two functioning wholes, so that part-self acts as the same self.

An Auschwitz doctor could, through doubling, not only kill and contribute to killing but **organize silently**, on behalf of that evil project, an entire self-structure (or self-process) encompassing virtually all aspects of his behavior...

The Nazi doctor knew that he selected, but did not interpret selections as **murder**. One level of disavowal, then, was the Auschwitz self's altering of the **meaning of murder**; and on the other, the repudiation by the original self of anything done by the Auschwitz self.

Indeed, disavowal was the life blood of the Auschwitz self... Doubling can include elements considered characteristic of **psychopathic character impairment**; ... Doubling may well be an important psychological mechanism for individuals living within any **criminal substructure**.

In *Doubling*, one part of the self "disavows" another part. What is repudiated is not reality itself – the individual Nazi doctor was aware of what he was doing via the Auschwitz self - but the meaning of that reality... The SS doctor – deeply involved in the stark contradictions of the "schizophrenic condition" lay in **the idea of doing constructive medical work within a slaughterhouse**.

From *When Healing Becomes A Crime* by Kenny Ausubel.[48]

In a brief twenty years, the AMA came to dominate medical practice through brute financial force, political manipulation, and professional authority enhanced by rising public favor with "scientific" medicine. The AMA emerged as the supreme arbiter of medical practice, making binding pronouncements regulating even the most picayune details. American medicine surged forward as a profit-driven enterprise of matchless scope. By the time Dr. Morris Fishbein assumed the mantle of Dr. Simmons, who had himself started out as a homeopath, the AMA was at the helm of a strapping new industry flying the allopathic flag. The code word for competition was "quackery."

Laws control the lesser man.
Right conduct controls the greater one.
Mark Twain.

Incest

It's safest to play with infants and children

Circumcision of both sexes and all <u>genital blood rituals</u> are incestuous and an act of female power relations => a menstrual feminization of the tribal male child and tribal female child's inclusion in her matriarchal blood/flesh incorporated group identity.[49]

70% Pakistani marriages are first cousin consanguineous[50] and more-so in the Kashmir region. Inbreeding has caused vast cases of genetic abnormalities.

About 3% of Great Britain births are of Pakistani descent and 30% of the Pakistani children are born with genetic birth defects both physical and mental.[51,52]

Incest used to maintain familial blood purity in Collective Narcissism is not uncommon.[53] In the Middle East it was practiced in Ancient Egypt to historic Judaism where down thru the ages the Jews have over 130 genetic diseases.[54,55] The state of Rhode Island allows uncle/niece avunculate marriage as an exemption for the Jewish religion.

Justification for child abuse stands on a rickety ethical framework that supplants immorality with a trans-morality.[56] The damaged internal child lives on for a lifetime.

Monteleone

Regardless of traumatic event, angst from genetic condition or any other multitude of factors the basic Abused to Abuser Cycle is similar. When a society incorporates abuse there is no family or social support. Monteleone noted:[57]

Sexual abuse in childhood appears to increase the risk for later sexual aggression, probably for the more severely traumatized children. Studies of sex offenders have revealed that many began their activities in mid-childhood after being sexually molested. Boys who are physically and sexually abused, unsupported in disclosing the abuse, and socially rejected are more likely to become delinquent or criminal than boys from supportive families. Many adult sex offenders may have been sexually abused in adolescence even before puberty.

Although the limited research cannot reliably predict who will become abusive, there is ample evidence of the damaging influence of abuse. While little direct evidence exists for an intergenerational transmission of sexual abuse, the complex traumatic components of child maltreatment are clearly associated with the behavioral symptoms, especially the physical and sexual aggressiveness of abused children.

Susan Forward, in *Toxic Parents*, wrote:[58]

With nothing and no one to judge them against, we assume them to be the perfect parents... The only way emotional assaults or physical abuse can make sense to the child is if he or she accepts responsibility for the toxic parents...

When you're young, our godlike parents are everything to us...

No matter how toxic your parents may be, you still have to deify them... There are two central doctrines in this faith of godlike parents: 1) "I am bad and my parents are good." 2) "I am weak and my parents are good," these are powerful beliefs that can outlive your physical dependence on your parents. These beliefs keep the faith alive; they allow you to avoid facing the painful truth that your godlike parents actually betrayed you when you were most vulnerable...

There are many parents whose negative patterns of behavior are consistent and dominant in a child's life. These are the parents who do harm... Many of the time-honored techniques that have been passed down from generation to generation are, quite simply, bad advice masquerading as wisdom.

There are parents whose negative patterns of behavior are consistent and dominant in a child's life. These are the parents who do harm. As difficult as it may be to believe, battered children accept the blame for the crimes perpetrated against them just as surely as verbally abused children do.

Sexual or physical abuse can be so traumatic that often a single occurrence is enough to cause tremendous emotional damage.

You are not responsible for what was done to you as a defenseless child! You are responsible for taking positive steps to do something about it now.

Universality of Incest

Again, spirituality is, theology explains, religion practices. Theology is expressed in mythological language. Religious practice takes a mythic story and develops it into a *Sacred Contract*. These Sacred Contracts, based on myth-working, do not always prohibit incest.

Besides parental incest, other forms of incest that appear in mythology include, in part, sibling, cousin, and niece/uncle incest as they are in Genital Play. Though niece/uncle marriage is illegal in America, a Jewish exception emulating the marriage of Abraham and Sarah, exists in the State of Rhode Island.[59]

When thinking of incest, a person first thinks of an adult male with a minor female relative.[60] One rarely thinks that boys might also be used sexually by mothers. It is rare for a male child or even a grown man.

Robert Miller, recalled the details of mother-son sexual abuse while in treatment at the Veterans Administration for PTSD, and Miller's incredibly moving poetry has been published in *Collection of Tears*.[61] Again, furthering deMause in, *The Universality of Incest*, about the **two types of incest – Direct** and **Indirect**:[62]

> Two kinds will be considered: *direct incest*, overt sexual activity between family members other than spouses; and *indirect incest*, the providing of children by their parents to others in order for them to be sexually molested. There are two reasons why I believe indirect incest must be included in any definition of incestuous activity.
>
> First of all, arranging for children to have sex with other household members or neighbors is usually motivated by the child (child's mind) to be similar to direct incest.
>
> Secondly, clinical studies show that contemporary sexual abuse involves a parent or guardian, who, if not the direct perpetrator, covertly brings about the incident in order to satisfy their own incestuous wishes.

Ritual Genital Dismemberments link to **societal indirect incest**. Circumcision in Islam signifies the boy leaving the mother to be with another woman.[63],[64] She is, in essence, giving her son to another female member of the societal group. As for the young ladies in groups that practice Female Genital Mutilation, circumcision allows them to marry – the same for young men.

deMause references Kitahara's *A Cross-Cultural Test of the Freudian Theory of Circumcision* that states.[65]

Genital mutilation rituals are cross-culturally correlated with exclusive mother infant skin-to-skin sleeping arrangements, where the father sleeps separate, so the mother is likely to use the child incestuously

From deMause's *The Universality of Incest* and paraphrasing including examples of incestuous habits – with the last five paragraphs are direct quotes:

As an adult, the pedophile must have sex with children in order to maintain the illusion of being loved, while at the same time dominating the children as they themselves once experienced domination, repeating actively their own caretaker's sadism.

The pedophile uses the child... for gratification and also as an object for sadistic aggression. ...

The pedophile's sexual targets are interchangeable and an active pedophile often seduces hundreds of children in his or her life. Adults who molest children have extremely powerful punitive superegos and are often highly religious.

Originally, male analysts regarded accounts of incest as wishful fantasies. Some had the opinion that incest did not present a problem. They considered the Incest Taboo that is common in all societies to be functionally effective.

Female analysts better understood the seriousness of incest and reported accounts of their child patients.

Many children were forced to handle their parent's genitals. Both parents gave daughters to male family members and friends for sexual purposes.

Incest statistics are probably higher than reported because high probability populations have not been well surveyed. These include incarcerated criminals, prostitutes, institutionalized children, psychotics and those who refuse to be questioned.

Memories prior to age five are usually suppressed, and half of reported molestations, with a fifth of reported rapes, are committed by those under age eighteen. Incidence would likely be higher where many societies are just beyond the Infanticidal Child Rearing Mode and use children for emotional needs. Using children for sexual purposes is also common in the Far, Middle and Near East., through the Qu'ran according to their age standards of when maturity begins (which is different for other religious groups).

As girls in the Middle East are considered worth less than boys, it has been reported that their incestuous use during childhood is even more prevalent. One report found that four out of five Middle Eastern women recalled having been forced into fellatio between the ages of 3 and 6 by older brothers and their relatives.

Arab women, of course, are often aware that their spouses prefer having sex with little boys and girls to having sex with them. Their retribution for the men's pedophilia comes when a girl is about 6, when the women of the house grab her, pull her thighs apart and cut off her clitoris and sometimes her labia with a razor, thus usually ending her ability to feel sexual pleasure forever.

Cliteroidectomy – like all genital mutilations of children is, of course, an act of incest motivated by the perversions of the adults who perform the mutilation...

Mothers who attack their daughter's genitals with knives are as incestuous as fathers who rape them.

Since genital mutilation is one of the most widespread child-rearing practices, its presence alone makes incest a universal practice – despite our habit of denying its sexual motivation by terming it a Rite of Passage or a Puberty Rite. Also, the sexual excitement of the adults attending the mutilation is overlooked, even when – as in Siwa – the mother masturbates the male child prior to mutilation, or when – as in Morocco – prostitutes regularly attend the mutilation in order to relieve the sexual tensions generated, or when – as in Australia – the mutilation is followed by a group rape.

The mutilation of children's genitals is such an important need in humans that whole religions and state systems have been founded upon the practice. Yet when scholars attempt to explain why almost everyone since the beginning of recorded history has massively assaulted the genitals of their children, they assiduously deny that it is a sexual perversion or that those who do it ever mean any harm to the children.

Maternal incestuous behavior with Female Genital Mutilation correlates to the masculine dominated incestuous social behaviors of 19th century British medicine that initiated, with the aid of American physicians, genital mutilation of both sexes.

Again, to reinforce, British doctors used to prescribe child sex to males with depression, impotence and venereal diseases.[66] Incest is predominant in emotionally dishonest societies. Dishonesty makes it difficult for the child to set boundaries and an inability to form adult relationships.[67]

Emotional Incest

Emotional Incest is a type of covert incest. Most do not recognize or admit victimization. Genital Dismemberments is a form of Emotional Blackmail, and forces the child to live in codependency. The parent uses the child for self-worth and definition. It permanently transfers power from the child, regarding bodily integrity, to the parent and society in the generational cultural system of abuse.

Freud, Hitler, and Stalin were their mother's Little Prince's, possible maternal codependent relationships could have been from maternal emotional incest.

Freud was his own first patient which may have led him to discover the Oedipus Complex, with its feminine counterpart, the Electra Complex.

Patricia Love in *The Emotional Incest Syndrome* stated:[68]

> To a large degree, our parents determined which parts of the self we were allowed to keep. Some of us were allowed to have needs, but not to be independent. We were catered to and indulged, but kept immature. Some of us were allowed a great deal of freedom, but not to have need. We were allowed to wander at will around the neighborhood, but were not given enough comfort and reassurance. Some of us were allowed to develop our talents, but were asked to repress our needs and emotions. We grew up to be compulsive achievers to hide an inner sense of inadequacy. To a greater degree than other children, we were not allowed to be whole. In exchange for love and a position of privilege in the family hierarchy, we had to give up a large portion of the self.

Circumcision presents a physical forever being. Pathology continues with being subjugated to the role of being responsible for parental self-gratification, safety, security, and well-being.

When the child matures and they themselves marry with children, they now assume the parental role in a Transgenerational never-ending cycle of abuse. If abusive habits continue and spread, working themselves into culture then the expansion is Socialization to Acculturation.

Emotional Incest may take many forms in a culture that accepts genital assaults on their children. deMause in an early edition exemplified:[69]

> *If I blow myself up and become a martyr, I'll finally be loved by my mother*
>
> That is what Palestinian terrorists say. They aren't looking for political change; they're looking for love. Love from Allah, yes – but really love from their parents. Palestinian mothers say they are raising martyrs, and pick which son should kill himself for her and never leave her. And as the terrorists strap their bombs on, they imagine they'll get the love they missed all their lives. How can mothers of martyrs say things like, "I was happy he blew himself up. Now he'll always be with me"?

Psychohistory

Lloyd deMause's book *Foundations of Psychohistory* documents generational abuse caused by: a) the psychosexual unified group, b) the effects of the group's abuse on the individual, and, c) the individual's subsequent responses back to the group.

Summarizing and commenting on deMause, not quoting:[70]

Psychohistory is the science of historical motivation. It interprets history, using psychoanalytical methods, for causes of historical events. It is normal and healthy for a person and community to organize existence in a structured environment so that life may be better for all.

Final outcomes are unique to each individual, community and culture. Sex is tied to social control. Basic motivations are the same with serial predators and religious ritual: power, control, and authority for domination, through manipulation out of selfishness.

Obtaining macro-social psychosexual cohesion in primitive society, the customs, mores, and rituals are centered on the reciprocal social functions of the sexes. The macro-social is the entire social that includes all sub-groups.

Each sub-group is a micro-social. The feminine function is procreation and taking care of offspring. The masculine function is to provide for the mother-child unit. This created two societies. The feminine is the internal central core. Mircea Eliade termed this the *Concept of the Center*.[71]

The masculine is the external periphery, surrounding the center. Primitive social rituals for the female stress the moon with menstruation. The social structure, for cohesion, needs controlling and protecting feminine reproduction.

Masculine penile rituals were often designed to mimic the trials and tribulations of the feminine, such as menstruation and birthing, thus creating empathy between men and women. Purely male rituals for the social purpose do not attack the penis – even though men's rituals often include odd behaviors such as object implantation for female stimulation.

deMause explains what cults do to children. These are micro-social forms of abuse because the cults deMause refers to, here, are sub-groups within the social. The children are often kept in cages, boxes, and coffins as womb symbols. Some are beaten and tortured; made to eat feces and drink urine and blood; eat food off adult genitals, forced to cannibalize; and sometimes are disemboweled and dismembered as the adults reach orgasm.

In these sadistic activities, some perpetrators are acting in regression and fear of reality, attempting to relive their own past trauma and relieve the anxiety caused by that trauma. The ritual is a delusional attempt to absorb the child's essence – to reclaim the power the perpetrator felt they lost as a child under similar conditions. Their actions are a literal acting out of what happened to them.

Cult abuse includes penetration of infants vaginally, anally, and orally. One common cult ritual is the Sacrificial Rebirth Ritual that may include a genital modification, as is the multi-faceted meanings with Jewish male circumcision. Children abused through sexual ritual are more psychologically symptomatic than those not sexually abused through ritual. Psychotherapists treating these children have had death threats and vandalism – as some opposing circumcision.

When infants and young children are abused in the preverbal state, they are amnesic. Preverbal memories are stored in the amygdala where our deepest fears reside. This is where sleep-terrors originate. The indescribable monster after you during sleep. *Sleep Terror Disorder*. When in touch with these night monsters, we do not act as our normal selves and the stored memories are, as deMause termed them, *alters*.

Declarative memory starts around three to four years old as we become verbal and when memory is now stored in the hippocampus. This is where *nightmares* originate. In social groups deMause termed the declarative memory as the basis of our *social alter*. Quoting deMause:[72],[73]

A group-fantasy, then, is produced by a collection of social alters as an agreement by groups of people to pool their traumas in a *Delusional Social Construction*.

Social alters have four main characteristics. They are:

1) Separate neural memory modules that are repositories for traumatic events and accompany feelings frozen in time.

2) Organized into dynamic structures containing a different set of goals, values, and defenses than the main self that help prevent the traumas and resulting despair from overwhelming the one's life.

3) Split off by a senseless wall of denial, depersonalization, discontinuous of affect and dis-ownership of responsibility that is maintained in collusion with others in society who have similar alters to deny

4) Communicated, elaborated, and acted out in group-fantasies embedded in political, religious, and social institutions.

Grooming

Before the term Grooming became associated with grooming a child for sexual abuse, the term Grooming was associated with coaching, mentorship, and preparing a person for leadership.

Grooming is making the appearance of normalizing inappropriate behavior between an adult and a minor. Groomers build their relationship on emotional connections building trust. Women, children and the young are more susceptible on their types of suggestion. Victims may be sexually abused, exploited and trafficked. Anyone can be a groomer no matter their sex, age or race.

Sexual Grooming means actions and behaviors used to attain emotional connections with a child and even the minor's family. The motive is to lower the child's inhibitions, and when present the family of the child to lower their inhibitions to, and for, sexual abuse.

Grooming can happen in any setting be it: online, in person or by any other means of communication. Children who are groomed may have mental health issues, including anxiety, depression, post-traumatic stress, and suicidal thoughts.

Men have committed suicide over their circumcisions. Well over 14% to 25% of circumcisions involving both sexes have lifelong deformations – besides the mutilation itself.

Paraphilia

Paraphilias are persistent recurrent sexual fantasies, urges or behaviors of marked intensity involving objects, activities, or even situations that are atypical in nature.

There are 8 paraphilic disorders: exhibitionistic, fetishistic, frotteuristic, pedophilic, sexual masochism, sexual sadism, transvestic, and voyeuristic.

Concentration on the object of their affection may be on a non-consenting partner or child. Holmes in Profiling Violent Crime wrote:

> There are adults who regard children as sex objects and as somehow deserving of exploitation as objects. For the person with such a mind-set, there is nothing wrong with sexually assaulting children. In fact, many child abusers apparently believe that children pursue adults for sex – an interesting rationalization that negates the child's personal responsibility. From this perspective, the child is the cause, the prime mover: the molester is the victim.

Kitahara states:[74] **Genital mutilation is always a punishment for growing up, is – rather a self-punishment for real maternal incest for which the children blame themselves.**

Neumann, in *The Great Mother* observed:[75]

She perpetually demands the blood of men.

Ritual Violence

The most powerful thing a society can do
Is to have others adopt their religious ritual

Humans are a predator species. Many rituals, including Genital Dismemberments are violent predations. Rituals are social enactments to control behavior. All rituals contain a *death motif* in one way or another and simulate life.

Ritual simulates all things in daily life, not just an African – Pre-Dynastic Egyptian - Hebrew circumcision, Catholic Mass, or Islamic Call to Prayer. It occurs each time one goes to a classroom, work, or vacation. When one finishes, whatever it is, they leave a different person from what is gained – a Life/Death/Life Cycle. But religious type rituals are different in that they occur in a mystic timed event.

How much are our decisions driven by social pressures, emotional blackmail, and guilt? Does a people's and a culture's varied behaviors as circumcision, a blood ritual, teach fear, distrust, learned helplessness and victim-consciousness, a self-defensive form of aggression, host and a "monkey-see-monkey-do" form of predation?

Purpose of Ritual

Rituals are repeated acts performed with symbolic value. They bond groups of people into a community, apart from other communities. They create an "us and them" mentality.

Social rituals are usually part of religion or simple tradition. Ancient rituals were designed to ensure survival. In a more complex society, people adapt to the same contingencies in a more complicated way.

Circumcision, i.e. Genital Dismemberments, are a mock human sacrifice and is, in essence, a *Partial Human Sacrifice*. They are social blood bonding rituals evolved from Full Human Sacrifice. In them a person "dies" to his or her individual nature and is "born" as a member of the group: the feminine, the ancient Wise Woman's, Life/Death/Life Cycle.

Order

Ritual act attempts to magically provide order in areas of perceived chaos. Our primal fear is that the interests of nature are somehow opposed to mankind. For humans, forms of order seem to ensure success.

Ritual is a method of ordering the hunt, or the timing of a proper harvest. Seasonal horticultural festivals – spring fertility and fall harvest – are rituals that are tied to the cycles of the moon. Sun rituals also exist for the depth of winter's darkness and the height of summer's light. In it all is the implication that humanity and its survival are the ultimate good and not to be questioned.

Circumcision's myth is Sarah did not reproduce until Abraham's circumcision, tying it to fertility and reproduction.

Joseph Campbell suggests that human sacrifice may have evolved from horticultural ideologies that in turn originated as survival rituals:[76]

Myth and rites referring to the mythological age, when the great mythological event took place that brought both death and reproduction into play and fixed the density of life-in-time through a chain reaction of significantly interlocked transformations, belong rather to the world system of planters than to the shamanistically dominated hunting sphere. Whenever such myths are found in a hunting society, acculturation from some horticultural or agricultural culture center can be supposed.

Power, Control, and Authority

Those who advocate ritual think power over nature and other people is necessary for survival, and that authority belongs to those who control both. In primitive cultures, genital rituals serve as a test of membership and loyalty to the tribe. It establishes group cohesiveness through blood, fear, and loathing for the purpose of bonding individuals together against perceived common external enemies.

From Dr. Catherine Bell, Emeritus Professor of Religious Studies; Santa Clara University, California:[77]

> The orchestrated construction of power and authority in ritual, which is deeply evocative of the basic divisions of the social order, engage the social body in the objectivation of oppositions and deployment of schemes that effectively reproduce the divisions of the social order,
>
> In this process such schemes become socially instinctive automatisms of the body and implicit strategies for shifting power relationships among symbols…
>
> Culture uses ritual to control by means of sets of assumptions about the way things are and should be.

Domination and Destruction

Once leadership and social identity are firmly established, rituals pit one group competitively against another in activities such as sports to war.

Rituals also attempt to mediate the guilt of humanity's destruction – killing and taking from nature – against the perceived positive value of humanity's continuance.

Prayers offered for animals killed in the hunt, or thanking the gods for a victory over enemies killed in war, represent an attempt to assuage nature's anger and mitigate man's guilt. They communicate an implied hope of forgiveness for having taken life.

The goal of ritual is acknowledgement of survival through domination. And, ritual itself sets domination of self and society's inter relationships. Bell stated:[78]

> Ritual mastery is itself a capacity for, and relationship of, relative domination…
>
> Binary oppositions almost always involve asymmetrical relations of dominance and subordination by which they generate hierarchically organized relationships…
>
> Fairly standard understandings involve the positive notion of "influence" on the one hand and the negative notion of "force" on the other.

Manipulation

Through ritual, people address the properties of nature they desire to control. Symbolic gestures, and objects are used, to represent the desired quality of nature, or a portion of the actual natural object can be used.

Sometimes the people dress and make images of themselves as if they are the object. What is done to, and with, the object explains man's intended manipulation of others and nature. Bell says:[79]

> Ritual practices never define anything except the terms of the expedient relationships that ritualization itself establishes among things, thereby manipulating their relationships.
>
> What is distinctive about ritual is not what it says or symbolizes, but that first and foremost is does things: ritual is always a matter of "the performance of gestures and the **manipulation of objects**.

Ritual as an Outlet for Violence

Some rituals are often violent social acts designed as outlets for violence. They mimic the violence considered necessary for controlling, directing, using, and justifying social behavior. From Bell:[80]

> Hence, ritualization is central to culture as the means to dominate nature and the natural violence within human beings. Although ritual (=culture) is the necessary repression of this violence (= nature), culture is still dependent upon the energy of aggression as well as its restraint...

Shifting Attack from Nature to Humanity

Ritual was directed toward controlling nature. But once nature ceased to be seen as a threat because immediate survival issues were resolved through more advanced hunting techniques and an increase in agricultural sophistication, many rituals were abandoned. Emphasis then turned to creating internal tribal hierarchy and external exclusivity.

Established leaders devised new rituals to maintain their positions of power. Some rituals changed and new ones were added, but all elements of ritual remained – power, control, and authority for domination out of selfishness.

Genital Dismemberments of children, require parents to sacrifice the genitals of their child in the mock-death ritual to earn the parents good standing in the social body, the seal of approval of religious leaders or medical professionals as "devoted," responsible parents.

If anthropologists looked at this mechanism from outside the system, such as in an ancient tribe it would be thought of as a "pledge of allegiance" or a "loyalty oath."

The Inevitability of Change

Rituals have changed and will continue to change. Yet, the message is still the same – success for the unified groupmind whichever manner the members imagine will make success possible. Dr. Joyce Brothers stated:[81]

> You can't make your kids not reinvent the wheel.

In the 1960's the Catholic Church allowed the Mass to be performed in the local language. Before that, the Church required the use of ancient languages; Latin, Greek, and Hebrew. Reason for language change is to increase communications and attendance. From Bell.[82]

> (Rituals) demonstrate that collective effervescences do not so much unite the community as strengthen the socially more dominate group through a "mobilization of bias."

Circumcisions and Group Identity

Ritual change is clear when observing puberty rites in neighboring cultures in the islands of Southeast Asia. The rituals are basically the same, but with subtle differences among tribes. Each tribe considers its own puberty rites "normal" and "proper" and the other's variations "odd" and "improper." Though purpose and meaning of changes that developed in the puberty rites were surely obvious to the participants at the time, the origin cannot be documented.

Circumcision gives group identity, fulfilling the urge for belonging. Thus "belonging" itself establishes an "us and them" mentality and a bias against outsiders is established. Punishing nonconformity reinforces group identity. In certain Muslim subcultures, a girl may be killed for just holding hands with a non-Muslim boy. Bell explains:[83]

> To approach cultural rituals as rooted in purely psychological conflicts is to see ritual as an oppression inherently necessary to society, which is defined in turn as the repression of the individual.
>
> Ritual structure is totally repressive instead of channeling violence, the order of ritual completely denies it.

Alternatives to Ritual

Catherine Bell stated there are only two alternatives for dissenters of social ritual. They appear to give it a **"no win"** situation for the weak of heart and mind. She wrote:[84]

> The only real alternative to negotiated compliance is either total resistance or asocial self-exclusion.

Inherent in either alternative is a problem. In total resistance, he'll be accused of being *anti-social*. If he chooses asocial self-exclusion he will be diagnosed with a *Schizoid Personality Disorder*.

The societal apocalyptic vision is forced upon the child

Anthropological

I Be, You Be, We Be

Acculturation

Some children do not survive adult entertainment

From our inner selves, reaching out and interacting with others, we develop social psychologies and ways to create cultural bonding. We establish social bodies with unique group: identities, countries, schools, families, and, gangs, to name a few.

Celebrating diversity is good and fine, but some things that knits us together into groups can also be used to separate us into hostile camps.

Some bonding activities can border on abuse. We accept abusive behavior as normal within our groups, only because we have become inured to the inherent violence due to historically agreed-upon social, moral, and legal codes of conduct.

Social rituals are repetitious and ever-changing due to each generation's existing power relationships. Changes may result in explanations for the ritual, or the way the ritual is performed, but the ritual – however explained or performed – must always take place because it establishes the seat of social power, control, and authority.

All societies integrate violence and aggression into socially sanctioned outlets. Most notably are competitive sports - strikingly, the apogee of the culture itself – before its downfall.

Violence can also be experienced vicariously through film and theater. Some rituals themselves may be violent and create harm through Munchausen behavior. Genital Dismemberment rituals create a *Cultural Post-Traumatic Attachment* that leads to a *Cultural Repetition Compulsion*.

Two basic biological functions perceived as *suffering* and *violent primal wounds* are menstruation and childbirth. Men attempt through ritual, often through matriarchal establishment, to emphasize with women or to undo women's pain and suffering in stoic manly silence.

Suffering, even if self-inflicted, can be used to elicit sympathy or worn as a badge of courage. This is one reason suffering enters ritual. *Genital Dismemberments are Feminizations of the tribal male and of the tribal female the inclusion to dominance within the matriarchy both within blood relations and the power of menstruation.*

Male initiation rites do not permit expressions of weakness. Returning back to the chapter on Islam, Joseph Campbell illustrated shared suffering in ritual during the Native American Plains Indians male ritual of Vow to the Sun where men would chant: *We must suffer as women suffer.*

Again, Campbell explains that: *Man doesn't enter life except by woman, and so it is woman who brings us into this world of pairs of opposites and suffering.*[85]

Transgeneration
Sometimes we choose to suffer alone,
Sometimes we choose to make others suffer with us

Transgeneration is when individual habits grow into local and regional patterns of behavior. At the initial stage, practices are not yet officially sanctioned in a culture or integrated into a country's social conscious, so they do not have legal protection. However, covert legal sanction exists when an act is against the law and proscribed by religion, and there is failure to apply the law and prosecute the behavior.

Abuses of all types are a result of repetition compulsion. Re-inflicting trauma on oneself or passing it on to another is an attempt to resolve the anxiety created by the initial trauma.[86] Battered girls, as women, often marry violent husbands; and, adult children of alcoholics often marry drinkers.

Goldman showed that a male circumciser is attempting to resolve his own circumcision by now playing the role of attacker.[87,88] Striking out at the young is transference of unresolved adult conflicts.[89] In this way children become social prey in an ongoing transgenerational cycle of violence and abuse.

Using a specialized agent transfers parental power to the social order, allowing the parent as well as society, non-responsibility through denial, deferral, deflection, and deceit. However, circumcisions of both sexes demand explanation because they cross physical boundaries.

The quest for perfection in the child stems from the parent's concern about adult perfection. From this parental perception, the elect transfer the general concept of human imperfection to the younger generation so that they may establish, maintain and enforce social mores.[90]

Transgenerational transmission of unresolved conflicts may come from parental feelings, including but not limited to: a miserable existence, insignificance, loneliness, abandonment, rejection, insecurity, and/or a need to belong.[91]

Attempts to resolve distress, where there is high dependence on others, involves a special anointing of self and society. Anointing includes special claims of authority, justification for physical punishment, identification in pain, inhibition of dissent, lack of accountability for the parent, a ritual agent, and the excuse of a *social right*.[92]

Ritual attempts to transform the initiate into society's vision of what is necessary for him or her to become an accountable member in good standing. Mystical traditions in social ritual often rely on history, theology, and religious practice.

Traditions often displace proper ethics allowing actions that would otherwise not occur. Ancient tribes used a specialized shamanic agent to perform rituals.

***Once you give up your integrity,
the rest is a piece of cake.***
J. R. Ewing. *Dallas.*

Socialization
**Genital Blood Rituals derive from the feminine
in menstrual, child birth, and death symbolism**

Socialization into the existing culture is **enculturation**. Enculturation is through **communal reinforcement** by repeating the societal values and norms to the child regardless of the lack of evidence to support society's position.

Introjection occurs when such behaviors become unconsciously accepted in the child's personality. Introjection is internalization of identification with parental figures and other aspects of the child's known world. Introjection is often accompanied with defense mechanisms for coping. **Coping** mechanisms are forms of denial, self-deception, and deferral, and are, as well, essential in ritual.

Group Dynamics

Group Dynamics involves behavior to current events. This behavior differs according to the individual's response to the local group. To achieve a new agreement the barriers of prejudices, expectations, ideology, theology, religious, and, control must be overcome. This can give rise to social constructionism which creates a perceived reality.

The new reality birthed in **social constructionism** is an invention of the culture that eventually appears obvious and as natural knowledge. This then established a consensus reality that is the reality the group or culture wishes to believe.

Peer Pressure

Peer Pressure imposes the group norm on individuals and requires people to conform. Peer Pressure works when opinion leaders prevail. Currently, this process is used to create the false demand for circumcision as a cure for AIDS. Many attempts to medically instill circumcision have been successful, but *all have been proven false*. The AIDS quest for circumcision is no exception as it is now in the past,[93] and the new excuses are arising with others circling back.

Groupthink

Groupthink occurs when people intentionally go along with what they think is the group opinion. Groupthink leads to improper and non-logical decisions. Groupthink uses the need for people to belong with others.

Symptoms of Groupthink include: a) illusion with invulnerability from unity, b) unquestioned belief, c) group rationalizations, d) stereotyping of opponents, e) self-censorship, f) direct pressure to conform, g) self-appointed guardians.

Groupthink creates *communal reinforcement* by repeating their assertions even if he cannot be proven.

Communal (Collective) Behavior

Communities reinforce *collective behavior* by instilling fear. The basis of all medical claims for Genital Dismemberments is fear. Medicine's fear is in not being dominant over Patient Preference. Patient's fear is being abused. Medicine thus needs to whip up **Collective Fear**.

Structuration

The overall method used is *Structuration* which is repeating the position of leaders with implied special knowledge who set the rules for others to live by. These people are acting as the public's **Social Agent**.

Institutionalization

The overall result of both sides is *Institutionalization*: As an example, are those who advocate circumcision want to continue and expanding its use, while those who oppose circumcision want to instill the fact that cutting children's genitals is truly improper behavior.

Social Norm

Once Genital Dismemberments (circumcisions) are established as a Social Norm it becomes easily enforced. Violations of norms are punished, even if it is only through social shunning. Violators are thought to be eccentric and alternatives are not acknowledged.

Circumcision is not the sole cause for the Abuser to Abused Cycle with its attending emotional responses. Circumcision adds to the numbers of dysfunctional people who reside within the Cycle of Betrayal

Of all possible factors, humiliation appears to be one of the requisites for subsequent pathologic behavior.

The majority of known serial killers live in the United States of America. This is abstract statistical evidence that is, in part, misleading.

World law enforcement realizes the vast majority of countries do not document as well as the US because of inability. Politics may hinder. Once in Russia, serial killing was considered a decadent Western phenomenon.

As with other types of sexual crimes a token is taken. In Genital Dismemberments it is the tissue. Yet, the tissue is discarded so the token taken from the crime scene is the victim him and/or herself. Then every time there is contact, a remembrance and/or communication the token presents for perpetrator vicarious re-experience if desired.

Humiliating rejection of innate and normal sexual existence whether biologically induced or ritualized may be their stressor to action taken.

Twofold Cyclic Emotional Pathway

The Abused to Abuser Cycle is vibrant, not static. It is like the figure eight; one cycle on top of the other connected illustrating dominance. Fear is a forcibly suppressed emotion in Genital Dismemberments, though fear always exists to the victim class.

It may also be perceived as the two cycles being side by side as the sign for infinity suggesting an ever forward movement in generational abuse with the topic of circumcision.

As a spider web, all conflictual emotions are interconnected. When a strand is plucked, its music sings to all. It is alive; it is us. For illustrative purposes, this emotional pathway does not matter which comes first. It represents a Cycle of Abuse in backlash after backlash after backlash. Repetition Compulsion in a Way of Life.

Phase 1: Starting with some of the *Victim's* initial emotions to the abuse:

Disfranchisement from loss of privilege for immunity is realized.

Self-esteem is lowered.

Guilt is the mantle taken regarding the Self.

Shame is guilt's response in relation to others.

Ignominy is the perceived Self; branded, disgraced, debased.

Disgrace becomes the place of existence.

Humiliation is the living existence.

Envy of others formulates.

Resentment of others is envy solidified.

Desperation tries to reconcile Self existence.

Hopelessness despair is reality of things unchangeable.

Phase 2: Result are some *Perpetrator's* emotions in response to being a victim:

Distress arises from betrayal.

Torment is increased with recurrent distress.

Anger evolves in displeasure of one's condition.

Hate is a result created.

Hostility becomes activated.

Aggression follows from frustration.

Violence onto another is perpetrated.

Rage is uncontrolled violence.

Wrath is a violent fit of rage.

Abuse is enacted to completion.

Justification is hypothesized to formality.

Expression

Woody Allen has made a film career portraying body part loss neurosis from a Jewish motif from unreachable Pre-verbal traumatic unconscious memory. It is as if one can come to enjoy their neurotic tendencies. Deception is primarily structured.

Islamic neurosis is directed both outward and inward in tribal directed violence. It is as if the behavior stems from Verbal adult remembered conscious memory of the traumatic event, not pre-Verbal unconscious memory stored in the id.

According Herve Bertaux-Navoiseau, African genocides by circumcision tribes onto non-circumcising tribes has led to 11 of the past 12 tribal genocides.

There is no psychological religious pillow given the Christian to rest his fractured psyche. Circumcision is against their religion. Psychopathy may be enhanced and lean toward Cognitive Dissonance in both Pre-verbal and Verbal memory. When reading their Christian Testament, internal conflict arises. Suffering is silent.

A large percent of these men who have become serial killers have had a poor relationship with their primary maternal caretaker as children where she possessed a Punitive Personality Disorder often using religion as an excuse to abuse the child.[94]

Unseen Disturbed Behavior

Circumcision is not the sole cause for the Abused to Abuser Cycle with its attending emotional responses. Circumcision adds to the numbers of dysfunctional people who reside within this Cycle on the social level.

Historically, male circumcision is the result of social stress management away from full human sacrifice into partial human sacrifice where some form of sacrifice must be maintained in fertility symbolism. Female circumcision is the result of stress management of a different origin from genetic genital difference among females.

Unseen are those affected by botched circumcisions. 4%, 1 in 25, occur in the only pertinent study. Such instances must be reported at the time of occurrence for proper statistics but rarely done. Subsequent treatment(s) are never recorded which increase percentile.[95] Female circumcision is worse.

Also, unseen are medical statistical ploys to perpetrate the circumcision ritual they usurped from the shaman. Discarded in the front are those they deny as botches though truly are; and, discarded are evidences of botches that are diagnosed after initial discharge. Perimeters of discard depend on each survey. Jung stated:[96]

> Any theory based on experience is necessarily 'statistical;' that is to say, it formulates an 'ideal average' which abolishes all exceptions at either end of the scale and replaces them by an abstract mean. This mean is quite valid, though it need not necessarily occur in reality.
>
> The statistical method shows the facts in the light of the ideal average but does not give us a picture of their empirical reality. While reflecting an indisputable aspect of reality, it can falsify the actual truth in a most misleading way. This is particularly true of theories which are based on statistics.

The unseen can be mysterious. Repetition Compulsion is a common result as a reaction to a past traumatic event. It is attempting to take control of the demon.

Repetition Compulsion is the unconscious tendency of a person to repeat a traumatic event or its circumstances. This may take the form of symbolically or literally re-enacting the event, or putting oneself in situations where the event is likely to occur again. Repetition compulsion can also take the form of dreams in which memories and feelings of what happened are repeated.

Unseen, unrecognized, disturbed behavior of circumcised individuals can be correlated to unseen disturbed cultural behavior in mutilating societies. Steven Lukes in *Political Ritual and Social Integration* wrote:[97]

> [Ritual] helps define as authoritative certain ways of seeing society; it serves to specify what in society is of specific significance, it draws people's attention to certain forms of relationships and activities – and at the same time, therefore, it deflects their attention from other forms, since every way of seeing is also a way of not seeing.

An American Epidemic

Most cultures do not allow children to be perceived as victims. The following is paraphrased from Elaine Landau's *Child Abuse: An American Epidemic* on the effects of child abuse. Landau describes many unfortunate signs we see in our society from early childhood abuse, and by inference relates to circumcision of both sexes. Summarizing:[98]

> Sympathy is given to young victims of abuse yet as these children grow, anti-social behavior clinically presents. In frustration, an attitude of deserving what has happened to them may develop.

Silently suffering, victims of abuse are too ashamed and afraid to seek help. Hand in hand with physical abuse, emotional abuse is generational mirroring the parental child-rearing techniques.

Adolescents, as well as adults, are unable to remove themselves from destructive relationships. Emotional scars are often untreated because they are sub-clinically unseen, yet they last a lifetime.

It is important for victims of genital cutting to learn stress management, otherwise abuses will continue to be passed down from one generation to the other both individually and socially.

The symptoms of abuse are many and varied, specific to the individual: physical, emotional and impairment; paralyzing fear or separation from the parent; impaired personal development; feeling of shame and guilt; bed-wetting; low self-esteem; hostility and other disruptive anti-social behaviors; a sense of desperation or unresolved anger; involvement in gangs, drugs, prostitution and/or crime; a pathological uncertainty about self and the world; either a profound lack of empathy for others, or an exaggerated "search for love"; hopelessness; and suicidal and/or homicidal impulses.

Eliade, Mircea in, *The Myth of the Eternal Return,* wrote:[99]

For traditional societies, all the important acts of life were revealed 'ab origine', by gods or heroes. Men only repeat these exemplary and paradigmatic gestures 'ad infinitum.'

All rituals imitate a divine archetype and that their continual re-actualization takes place in one and the same atemporal mythical instant. However, the construction rites show us something beyond this: hence re-actualization of the cosmology.

Myth

There are many aspects to myth and each has their myriad of definitions. Interpretation of myth can focus on the following elements: Comparative Mythology, Functionalism, Euhemerism, Allegory, Personification and Myth-Ritual Theory

Two definitions, as excerpts on myth, may help the reader in brief mention: First by Lauri Honko. Second Jose Manuel Losada:[100],[101]

Myth, a story of the gods, a religious account of the beginning of the world, the creation, fundamental events, the exemplary deeds of the gods as a result of which the world, nature and culture were created together with all parts thereof and given their order, which still obtains.

A myth expresses and confirms society's religious values and norms, it provides a pattern of **behavior to be imitated,** testifies to the efficacy of ritual with its practical ends and establishes the **sanctity of cult.**

Myth is the oral, symbolic, evolutionary and apparently simple account (in the sense of a tale, a diegesis, or a series of narrative and representative actions) of an extraordinary experience or event with a transcendental and personal reference that shows social classification.

Considered, in principle, as bereft of historical testimony, myth is composed of a series of constant or invariable cultural semantic elements which can be reduced to themes, and is endowed with a conflictive (it invariably contains a trial or ordeal), functional character (understood as the transmission of common values and beliefs, and the provision of factual **schemata of rites and actions**) and etiological nature (expressing in some way a particular or universal cosmogony or eschatology).

Again, Mircea Eliade observed that during a ritual the person/group psychic being transfers to the time/place of the original ritual in which it is based – as circumcision. Joseph Campbell stated to the effect: *When you participate in a ritual you are participating in a myth.*

How To Take a Life Without Taking Life?[102]

1) **Remove the victim's meaning of existence and the genitals are part of it.**

2) **So too, taking away the perpetrators personal and professional livelihood.**

Circumcision homicides over 400 children of both sexes a year. The play-death game of genital blood rituals engaged in by malpractice Health Care Professionals and False Prophets of playing Deity "I am God" pontifications is extremely serious. Serial killers who kill their victim to the point of unconsciousness and then letting the victim resuscitate are playing: I=God. Edward Edinger wrote:[103]

> Now if any of those containers of one's psyche dies, one goes through a grief reaction because a piece of one's self dies at the same time. One has to take back that piece of one's own psyche from the person who has died, otherwise it will pull us into the grave,
> The same thing can happen when a person or object dies for us psychologically – *it doesn't have to be a literal death.* There's a psychological death when the projection that has been carried for us to drop off. A piece of ongoing life we were used

to has disappeared, and we are in effect dead until that missing piece of our psyche is recovered.

Desexualization is one of the main objectives of circumcision for both females and males. The Jewish tradition of circumcision stems back into Pre-Dynastic Egypt not in Mesopotamia's Babylon in conjunction to Pakistan and Iran.

In this many may possess Punitive Personality Disorder.[104] Sexual Sadist Rabbi Moses Maimonides in the 12th Century wrote in his Guide to the Perplexed wrote:

> The bodily pain caused to that member is the real purpose of circumcision. None of the activities necessary for the preservation of the individual is harmed thereby, nor is procreation rendered impossible, but the violent concupiscence and lust that goes beyond what is needed are diminished. The fact that circumcision weakens the faculty of sexual excitement and sometimes perhaps diminishes the pleasure is indubitable. For it is at birth this member has been made to bleed and has had its covering taken away from it, it must be indubitably weakened. The Sages, may their memory be blessed, have explicitly stated: It is hard for a woman with whom an uncircumcised man has had sexual intercourse to separate from him.
>
> The perfection and perpetuation of the Law can only be achieved if circumcision is performed in childhood... The parents of the child that is just born take lightly matters concerning it, for up to that time the imaginative form that compels the parents to love it is not yet consolidated.

Before learning what pathology looks like, a surgeon must know what normal tissues look like. The same pertains to ritual. Ritual deals with identity, moods and motivations.[105]   This includes identity in self and social images.

Circumcision creates a Brand Personality, a *social totem*, and that in turn is constructed in social requirements to belong, in to repeat, entering the same room from a different door => ***The Totem Penis and Totem Vulva***.

It can never be stressed enough that circumcisions are a form of ancestor worship in mock death ritual, a type of self and social deification. Jean-Paul Sartre observed: "Fascism is not defined by the number of its victims, but by the way it kills them."

It is imperative for people and society to see the humanity of children, adjust behavior, and cease the abuse of circumcision – a Genital Dismemberment that is a hallmark of a Lust Murder, and theologically belongs to goddesses.[106]

Every life is a march from innocence, through temptation, to virtue or vice. … Do not think you can fight corruption without while you let corruption fester within.
Lyman Abbott. *Problems of Life.*

Munchausen Complex

Mother binds Father; Father binds Mother; We are Spawn of their Argument

When someone calls for attention by *harming themselves*, it is called *Munchausen Syndrome* in honor of Baron Karl Freidrich von Munchausen who fictionalized his military and hunting exploits.

When one person *harms another* (usually someone under their care, such as an infant, child, or elder) and subsequently gains attention by becoming involved in their victim's medical treatment, it is called *Munchausen Syndrome by Proxy*. Sometimes they spread throughout the family and the social body.

The *Munchausen Complex* is a many faceted extensions within the Munchausen Syndrome and Munchausen Syndrome by Proxy.

Munchausen Syndrome (MS)

In 1951, Sir Richard Archer, an English physician, introduced the term Munchausen Syndrome.[107] Munchausen Syndrome is a mental disorder in which a person fabricates signs and symptoms of illness for attention and sympathy. Munchausen perpetrators are not hypochondriacs who actually think they are ill. A Munchausen patient knows their condition is false. They do not always clearly understand that their motivation is to obtain attention and sympathy of others.

According to the American Psychiatric Association Munchausen Syndrome is a form of Factitious Disorder.[108] *The Merck Manual* states:

> Commonly, there is an early history of emotional and physical abuse. Patients appear to have problems with their identity, intense feelings, inadequate impulse control, a deficient sense of reality, brief psychotic episodes and unstable interpersonal relationships. Their need to be taken care of conflicts with their inability to trust authority figures, whom they manipulate and continually provoke or test. Feelings of guilt and expiation are obvious.

Wounding for the Social Purpose

Wounding for social purposes can be performed by the person themselves onto their own bodies, but most often the actions are performed by a ritual expert, such as a shaman or physician onto the body of another community member.

Some forms of the Munchausen Complex may be minor, but other forms can become severe. Genital Dismemberments have taken too many lives and every one suffers deformity. For females the number of deaths most likely than not is much higher than that of the males.

Examples of wounding for social purposes that include children as well as adults, in part, include:

Flagellation	**Oral Modification**
Piercing	**Finger Amputation**
Tattooing	**Flesh Amputation**
Branding	**Trepanation**
Scarification	**Skeletal Deformation**

Teratophilia is a term that indicates an attraction to people with deformities.

Munchausen Syndrome by Proxy (MSBP)

In 1977, English pediatrician, Roy Meadow, defined Munchausen Syndrome by Proxy (MSBP).[109] MSBP occurs when the person, usually but not always mothers, seeking attention causes harm by manufacturing injury, illness, or disease in another person.

The perpetrators payoff is attention gained from involvement in treatment. This way they become the alter-patient. Most often MSBP involves a parent or caretaker harming a child under their care. The child is the means to an end.

The DSM-IV defines MSBP as a form of Factitious Disorder.[110] **MSBP is a crime with a victim.**

Health care providers, attorneys, social servants, and even courts are reluctant to believe that a mother would intentionally inflict harm on a child. Often professionals are so busy trying to find a proper diagnosis that they overlook the larger picture. Stopping abusive behavior is difficult even when the perpetrator undergoes long-term therapy.

Munchausen Syndrome by Proxy perpetrators are indifferent to the well-being of their victims who are usually infants and toddlers. Older children, adults, the elderly, and infirm may also be victimized. Children may become permanently deformed.

Common victim symptoms are diarrhea, vomiting, seizures, and respiratory failure. As with practitioners of Munchausen Syndrome who leave when confronted, the proxy perpetrator will take the victim elsewhere.

There are three types of Munchausen Syndrome by Proxy perpetrators: 1) help seekers, 2) doctor addicts, and, 3) active inducers.[111],[112]

1) **HELP SEEKERS** are often mothers who seek medical attention for their children in order to communicate their own anxiety, exhaustion, depression, or inability to care for the child. Case examples of help seekers include homes studded with domestic violence, marital discord, unwanted pregnancies, or single parenthood.

2) **DOCTOR ADDICTS** are obsessed with obtaining medical treatment for nonexistent illness in their children. The falsifications of doctor addicts consist of inaccurate reporting of history and symptoms. Such mothers believe their children are ill, refuse to accept medical evidence to the contrary and then develop their own treatment for the children. The children usually are older than six years and the [caretakers] are suspicions, antagonistic, and paranoid. These mothers tend to be distrustful and angry.

3) **ACTIVE INDUCERS** induce illness in children by dramatic methods. These mothers are anxious, depressed, and employ extreme degrees of denial, dissociation of affect and paranoid projection. Secondary gain for these mothers includes a controlling relationship with the treating physician and acknowledgment from medical staff as outstanding caretakers.

Another manifestation of MSBP, perpetrators will induce a condition to "heroically save" the victim thereby showing they are a concerned caretaker. Sometimes health care providers – including nurses of both sexes – do this.

This phenomenon may very well be a distinct category of Munchausen that should be redefined as ***Munchausen's Malignant Hero Syndrome***.

Diagnosing Munchausen Syndrome by Proxy is difficult and may be over-diagnosed. Support groups are available for those falsely accused of Munchausen Syndrome by Proxy. It is always possible that a caretaker has legitimate concerns about his or her child's health that are not being adequately addressed.

*Some people **wrongly prosecuted** for Munchausen Syndrome by Proxy have had children with **undiagnosed genetic defects**.*

The Munchausen Complex

Munchausen Syndrome and Munchausen Syndrome by Proxy are conditions involving harm to self, another, and/or others. When Munchausen behaviors extend and enter the greater picture of the social arena, all together they form a ***Munchausen Complex***.

The following individual designations, in part, within the Munchausen Complex are hereby put forward in this initial proposal.

Transgenerational Munchausen

Transgenerational Munchausen Syndrome is the passing of Munchausen Syndrome and Munchausen Syndrome by Proxy abuses to successive generations. The purpose is to feed the need of belonging through Attachment Seeking.

Transgenerational Munchausen is not fully acculturated. It is often, though not always, achieved through purposeful Cultural Imperialism.

TRANSGENERATIONAL MUNCHAUSEN is a Munchausen syndrome where generational abuse in family and social groups are a step toward socialization and acculturation.

Munchausen Syndrome in Social Transference

When abusive Munchausen behaviors manifest in a social context and becomes commonplace and acceptable, a social identity shift occurs through social transference. Transference is defined as the displacement of one's unresolved conflicts, dependencies, and aggressions onto a substitute object.

With Genital Dismemberments, the object is a specific part of the body, the genitals. Genital Blood Rituals are matriarchal originations through perceived sexual conflict.

A historic example mentioned earlier for Islam, and the same in recent years for Anglophone Christianity, is the habit of Genital Dismemberments, called circumcision, directly from the Jewish faith who themselves adopted it from elsewhere. It is practiced on both males and females.

MUNCHAUSEN SYNDROME IN SOCIAL TRANSFERENCE is the identity transference of the Self into a social group that practices forms of Munchausen behavior.

Munchausen Syndrome in Collective Transmission

Munchausen Syndrome in Collective Transmission is the transmission of destructive behavior, harmful ritual, condition, or simulation of disease whether physical or psychological or both, taken to clinical significance whether to a person or another person or group of persons.

The act involves transference of an identity into interpersonal, family, community, societal or cultural relationships. The act(s) often operate by deliberate transmission from one generation to subsequent generations of unresolved conflicts, dependencies, and aggressions, onto an object or an objectified human body part of unresolved issues, onto heirs and associates.

Actions become social mores – customs and conventions. Mores embody the fundamental collective views of a group. They are accepted without question and they give power to those who perform them within some kind of social ritual. Group Identity gives security through social cohesion and conformity.

As with other forms of Munchausen, Collective Munchausen includes a type of *wounding*, physically and/or psychologically. Wounding is usually, though not always, performed by a member of the group onto another.[113]

Abraham's circumcision story is an example. First Abraham circumcised his son, then he himself, then the rest of his clan, then slaves, and then followers. Genocidal.

MUNCHAUSEN SYNDROME IN COLLECTIVE TRANSMISSION extends Transgenerational Munchausen into a community, society, and/or a culture often within the context of social identity.

Collective Munchausen in Social Agency

Agency relationships involve a person called an Agent who acts for and represents another person called the Principal. The Agent acts through the authority transmitted to him/her by the Principal.

The fallacy for procedures as Genital Dismemberments on minors is the doctor is *not* the Agent of the parent as the principal, but the doctor is actually the Agent of the infant or child who is the Principal and who will become the **victim**.

Since the law does not allow or acknowledge any authority of Agency to minors or the mentally incompetent, the courts and law enforcement are the Agents of the infant, child, and the mentally incompetent when Collusive Abuse occurs or is about to occur.

MUNCHAUSEN SYNDROME IN SOCIAL AGENCY is the relationship between the "principal" who is the person with a primary legal agency, usually a parent or caregiver and another person; the "agent" who accepts "secondary agency," is usually a doctor of shaman who creates an act of abuse within social group behavior.

Munchausen Syndrome for Profit

Usually Munchausen motives are for attention, self-glorification, and adulation from others. Yet financial gain can be another motive. For Munchausen Syndrome for Profit to be a successful the endeavor must be perceived to be socially acceptable.

In many places where Female Dismemberments occur the women perform the ceremony and often the only 'job' they are allowed to have.

MUNCHAUSEN SYNDROME FOR PROFIT is 1) the fabrication of disease, physical or mental, or exacerbation of an existing medical condition by a person, often with a specialized agent such as an attorney or special interest group, to gain sympathy from others and/or society for financial gain; as well as, 2) non-monetary gain including values associated, in part, power, prestige, and employment security.

Collective Munchausen Syndrome for Profit

COLLECTIVE MUNCHAUSEN SYNDROME FOR PROFIT refers to social activities that involve abuse of a person or groups of persons for the motives of financial gain as well as other concepts of value including power, prestige, and employment security.

Genital Play

The child is not considered fully human, just an extension of the adult-Self, leaving way for fun and games, and if early enough the child would not remember.

Genital Play is a natural part of a healthy human body. In the womb, the fetus touches its genitals. This continues for comfort not sexual function. Genital Play and ritual have strong connections to sexual identity and life in the social community.

Some adults use children for their own sexual pleasure. Even Genital Dismemberments give pleasure for some adults and up until now have been used thusly based on religion through theology. Recently Genital Play has been secularized where humanity replaces a deity.

A child feels powerless when confronted by adult sexual attention. Memories of childhood sexual abuse make grown men and women cry even beyond 60 years later.

Child Abuse Through the Ages

Most abuses that become socialized begin at home with a child as the target. Abuse is passed down into succeeding generations often into society.

In *The Universality of Incest* Lloyd deMause discussed many examples of abusive Genital Play.

Some abuses have been defended through religious argument, though upon scrutiny are invalid, but some have melded into religious practices.

What is at play is often overlooked – self-deification of the perpetrator.

From deMause.[114]

China used to have a system of adopting children for incestuous purposes. *Their religion taught that the more partners a man acquired, the more **life force** he would have.* Also, a girl might be adopted to be the family son's wife, and a boy might be adopted to be a daughter's husband. Boy and girl prostitution was widespread as well as slaves and servants. There was also a system for older men to marry young boys who were often castrated, and they had gods of pederasty. Foot-binding of girls from all socioeconomic classes did not always include the big toe; it was left unbound for male sexual use. This penis-toe was used for anal stimulation of the male and for sucking on it. Boys adopted for sex were also foot-bound.

Ancient Japan also used child prostitution of both sexes. Temple prostitution was common. Boys were used in pederasty by samurai and priests, and to some the boys reached status. Royal incestuous marriage was encouraged for all ages. Incest was considered proper conduct. Some mothers masturbated their sons as if it was as common as toilet training. They thought it important to give him his first orgasm. It was not uncommon for sons to sleep with their mothers into their teens.

The degree of incest varied to family habits with the mother, as well as the children sleeping together. Some in Japan considered Oedipus problems negated because, in essence, the mother rejected the father and he went elsewhere for socially sexual relations.

Some cultural practices, including parts of India, persisted from ancient Zoroastrianism. In India both sexes were masturbated by their mothers. After age 5 the children were used for sex by extended family members, and referred to as "Little Wives." Uncle-niece and cross-cousin marriage were preferred and Sarai/Abram were from Ur of the Chaldees.

Children were prostituted by and with priestly authority by the Vedic Brahmins. Women were expected to kiss the genitals of the penis-god Siva's priests. The Indian epic Mahabharata states a 30-year-old man should marry a girl before she menstruates and a father who objects will go to hell.

In these societies, adult intercourse was considered polluted. The Baiga of India practiced parent and grandparent incest marriage with children. The Muria, who lived in some relatively isolated forested areas of India, sent their children to sex dormitories after age 5.

A covenant not to defend myself from force, by force, is void.
Thomas Hobbes. *Leviathan*.

Criminology

The psychological indicators of serial sexual predation
Are similar to those of religious genital blood rituals

REPORTING CHILD ABUSE: Monteleone wrote *Recognition of Child Abuse for the Mandated Reporter*. It is the main go-to reference for Reporters suspicions. Again:[115]

> *Child abuse involves every segment of society and crosses all social, ethnic, religious and professional lines. The definition of child abuse can range from a narrow focus, limited to intentional inflicted injury, to a broad scope, covering any act that adversely affects the developmental potential of a child. Included in the definition are neglect (acts of omission) and physical, or sexual injury (acts of commission) by a parent or caretaker. Intent is not considered in reporting abuse; **protection of the child is paramount**...*
>
> *The sex offender often pursues this practice as a career and will abuse many children over the course of time.*

Richard Dawkins in *The Selfish Gene* introduced the concept of the *meme*.[116] A meme is a social, psychological tool often used by humans to pass down cultural identity via imitation. Memes can be customs, language, music, dietary habits, catch phrases, fads, fashion, humor and circumcision.

In *Ritual Theory, Ritual Practice* Catherine Bell writes that ritual is motivated by five things: power, control, authority, manipulation, and domination.

The FBI agents who originated criminal profiling use the exact same five words and add one more: selfishness.

101

Criminologist, Colin Evans connects the dots between criminology and the repetitive nature of genital mutilation rituals.[117]

> Serial killers are usually creatures of habit; they find a method of destruction that works and stick to it.

Sexual Predation

Any empathy expressed by a predator for the victim is purely self-serving.[118]

Objectivation is the degradation of another person by perceiving him or her as an object as opposed to honoring him or her as a valuable human being.

This is a form of Dissociation that separates a person or group of persons from their fundamental humanity. Dissociation is integral to the perpetration of violence and abuse against others.

Assault and Battery with Attempt to Disfigure the genitals onto those who are of minor age is such a case, an example so obvious and unspeakable; therefore, read about it.

Transgender surgery is presently being forced onto society and children psychologically. But this text is to make one think, so it will use what is considered normal but in reality, is not so much different.

Reporting Child Abuse

Dr. James Monteleone wrote *Recognition of Child Abuse for the Mandated Reporter*. It is the main go-to reference for Reporters suspicions. To stress:[119]

Child abuse involves every segment of society and crosses all social, ethnic, religious and professional lines. The definition of child abuse can range from a narrow focus, limited to intentional inflicted injury, to a broad scope, covering any act that adversely affects the developmental potential of a child. Included in the definition are neglect (acts of omission) and physical, or sexual injury (acts of commission) by a aren't or caretaker.

Intent is not considered in reporting abuse; **protection of the child is paramount**... The sex offender often pursues this practice as a career and will abuse many children over the course of time.

Dismemberments is to perpetrate their social structure and themselves in their social hierarchy by making circumcision the social norm ritual, regardless of how that ritual affects themselves or their victims.

Again, as in serial killing, the object of Genital Dismemberment is power, control, and authority through manipulation out of selfishness. Acculturated Sado-Masochism.

Douglas and Olshaker stated.[120]

So, let's get this straight and state it plainly: It is my belief, based on several decades of experience, study, and analysis, that the overwhelming majority of repeat sexual predators do what they do because they want to, because it gives them a satisfaction they do not achieve in any other aspect of their lives, and because it makes them feel good, regardless of the consequences to others.

In that respect, the crime represents the ultimate in selfishness; the perpetrator doesn't care what happens to the victim as long as he gets what he wants. In fact, exercising this manipulation, domination, and control – and the infliction of pain and death are for him their ultimate expressions – are the critical factors in making him feel complete and fully alive.

Connie Fletcher in *What Cops Know* wrote about rape associated with inflicting pain. And circumcisions of both sexes are rapes.[121]

Rape is about anger, power, control, and the need to humiliate somebody. It's not sex driven. Many times, the rapist is also having consensual sex while he's going out raping…

Usually, it's not the sex that excites them; it's the sense of power they get over the victim. With some rapists, they're not there for the sex. They're there to inflict pain.

Motivational Cycle of Betrayal

The motivational process of most sexual crimes is circular and similar to a serial sexual offender's criminal ritual. It is a Cycle of Betrayal.

POWER > CONTROL > AUTHORITY > MANIPULATION > DOMINATION > SELFISHNESS

BETRAYAL

The cycle begins with a feeling of Betrayal which the perpetrator tries to mediate by obtaining and exercising *power*. Performing a power-based action is to effect *control* over them. A successful action that gives assumed authority gives the perpetrator a sense of *authority*. It also assumes a right to exercise influence over another person's life in order to fill a lack in the perpetrator's own inner self. The active component is *manipulation*. *Domination* is established by a successful *manipulation*. The act is perpetrated out of *selfishness*. If unchallenged, rule is established with maintenance assured. With success in the entirety of the procedure another Betrayal is then perpetrated.

This *Cycle of Betrayal* that begins with a Betrayal and ends with a Betrayal may be thought of as *Signatures Desire*. 76% of rapists were sexual abuse victims when young. The selfish motive that is almost universal is: *Because They Want To.*

If a victim's resentment is toward the father, aggression will most often be directed at males. If resentment is toward the mother, aggression will most often be directed at females. Again, circumcision of either sex has been described as a **mock-death ceremony**.[122],[123] The following concept of representation is derived from Douglas and Olshaker.[124]

> The victim is a representation. It is as if the American President of the United States society, and the male child represents the masculine. The intellectual overlay, especially to the Organized type is a cause.

The cause used as an excuse is a convenient justification. It is transference in Reason Avoidance so not to confront and deal with reality. There is often a dissociation of the perpetrator's parental figure to the same sex of the victim

The violent act is from a deep-seated inadequacy. To solve the problem of inadequacy the represented object must be defiled or eliminated. The male becomes an object and inferior.

Once the course of action is decided, the Organizer is calm and the internal conflict of stress is mostly eliminated... the offenders who get close and personal to their victim actually do not get emotionally involved. This dissociation maintains distance. Thus, they feel comfortable in the situations they are able to control.

There is no remorse or contrition. Everything is matter of fact. They know the difference between right and wrong. **Changing wrong to right changes the standards. This then makes the consequences non-consequential.**

The definition of sexual sadism is sexual arousal gained from inflicting pain and suffering on others. Sexual sadists are among the most destructive of all predators.

These predators focused on the goal and the process of inflicting pain and humiliation onto the victim, as rabbi Maimonides. They torture to inflict both physical pain and mental anguish. Sadism is highly symbolic and often hides behind the excuse of religion, often in sly self-deification.

The sadist's core fantasies are cemented by age sixteen. Sadists have no remorse or sympathy. The victim is depersonalized to object status. Killing is their apogee in obsessive control. *Piquerism* may also be a component.

There are two types of sadism: *minor* and *major*. **Minor sadism** involves partners who consent to bondage, discipline, spanking, and submission to degrading acts. **Major sadism** involves consenting partners, or non-consenting victims.

Psychopathology

Douglas and Olshaker state:[125]

When you've analyzed what should be the motive based on the crime scenario and that doesn't make sense, and you go through all the other "logical" ones and you can't make one of them fit reasonably, then you start looking into psychiatric territory.

All crimes have a motive; all crimes make sense according to some logic, though that logic may be a strictly internal one with no relationship to any "objective" logic. In many instances, a hidden sexual motive emerges, a motive that originates in fantasy,

Tragically, this motive of uncontrolled anger and the need for sexual domination doesn't always occur against strangers. Many sexual sadists are married or in ongoing relationships – totally self-involved narcissists.

Psychopathology involves three characteristics:
1) **Egocentricity**
2) **Lack of empathy**
3) **No remorse**

Narcissistic psychopaths feel they have special entitlement.[126]

As with serial killers, they have a system of destruction and bring that destruction to others. This permits, using and taking from others to enhance their status internally, monetarily, and socially.

Psychopaths lie. When caught, they make up other lies. This is seen in various rationalizations for circumcision. They restructure arguments as needed. Circumcision has been touted a remedy for many ailments and when disproved, they invent another excuse that is a never-ending cycle by repeating the first disproven excuse to a new generation.

The **Service Personality** appears humble, sensitive, profound. They say publicly what would be expected. Behind the scenes they laugh, joke, and brag.

Psychopaths are not emotionally attached to other people; they do not see others as valuable. Instead, they are attached to impersonal objects such as knives, blood, and human body tissue. **Their object possesses magical powers**. They use it almost like a magic wand.

The genitals, which possess natural, pleasurable, reproductive powers are made subservient to the psychopath's will. The natural genitalia are defeated by the "magical power" of the knife or any other instrument of choice. They will not change or stop. They are untreatable.

Douglas and Olshaker wrote:[127]

> This is really nothing but elementary butchery. We have long since learned that serial killers need nothing but will to commit whatever atrocities they want on a body.

They are willing to have someone else die for their selfish purposes, and that is one of the definitions of sociopathic behavior.

Based on my research and experience, there is no possibility of rehabilitating this type of individual. **If he is ever let out, he will kill again.**

The Child Molester

Circumcisions of both sexes is child molestation. Child molesters believe they do no wrong and even imagine that they improve their victim's lives. To stress, child molesters and serial killers share a same personality type. Their attack neutralizes their greatest threats first.[128] In the case of circumcision, the parent must be disarmed, usually with charm. One method of classifying child molesters separates them into two groups: 1: Preferential; and, 2: Situational.

The **Preferential Child Molester** seeks certain objects of affection be it age, race, sex and other factors that attracts.

The **Situational Child Molester** is where genital assaults reside. The Situational Molester has **4** sub-sets:
Morally Indiscriminate; Inadequate
Sexually Indiscriminate; Regressed

Genital mutilators mainly, but not always, fit the *Situational Child Molester*, subset *Morally Indiscriminate*.

Socialized Genital Dismemberments allow everyone to attend with their own particular quirk.

Manipulation

Lie to me, lie to me, tell me what I want to hear

What kind of mental programming has made us blind to the practice of Genital Dismemberments in the world – especially in modern industrialized countries?

It is in Power Relations.[129]

> **Power Relations** refers to relationships in which one person has, or a group of persons have, over another person, or group of persons, and is able to get the person or group of persons, to do what they wish whether by compelling obedience or in some less compulsive and even a more subtle way.

The Herd Mentality

Edward Bernays was often referred to as *The Prince of Puff* and *Baron of Ballyhoo* believed the common person was a member of the *Herd* of human existence, inferior, and are to be led, directed, controlled, and used by the *Elite* people of the world of which he considered himself to be.

Bernays stated:

> The conscious and intelligent manipulation of the organized habits and opinions of the masses is an important element in democratic society. Those who manipulate this unseen mechanism of society constitute an invisible government which is the true ruling power of our country. We are governed, our minds are molded, our tastes formed, our ideas suggested, largely by men we have never heard of. This is a logical result of the way in which our democratic society is organized.

Bernays was Sigmund Freuds nephew. He proudly applied his uncle's psychological discoveries to his knowledge as a WWI Propaganda Officer. In 1928 Bernays' *Propaganda*, the handbook was used by Joseph Goebbels, the director of Propaganda for the Hitler Nazi government.

He dubbed himself the Father of Public Relations. After the war he used his propaganda skills to fool the public into accepting his clients commercial, medical, and political products. Bernays coined the phrase *Big Think* for his shrewdly-veiled marketing practices including: publicity stunts, third-party authorities as doctor endorsements, national surveys, and product branding.

Bernays believed in *The Intelligent Few*. He paid his chauffeur he called Dumb Jack twenty-five dollars a week. Dumb Jack worked from 5:00 AM until 10:00 PM with a half day off every two weeks. *"Not a bad deal,"* said Bernays, *"but that's before people got a social conscious."*

THE BERNAYS EFFECT: the improper and successful manipulation of an individual, group, or the general public for power, control, authority and/or financial gain.

Again, **suggestibility** is **responsiveness to suggestion**. Those who initiate, perpetrate, and maintain ritual rely on suggestibility. The two types of suggestion are **direct** and **indirect**. People respond to both, but are generally predisposed to one or the other. The physically-inclined respond more to **direct suggestion**. Those emotionally-inclined respond more to **indirect suggestion**.

Suggestibility is fostered by three factors:

1) **Extension** – Bystanders get caught up in a movement.
2) **Intensification** – Individuals observe the opinion shared by the crowd
3) **Predisposition** – Universal sympathy to the opinion makes a similar response easier the next time.

These three reactions are reinforced by an authority figure's perceived superior power, leading to control due to awe or fear. The power may come from an individual – a parent, religious leader, physician, or a tribal elder – or society itself may act as the superior power.

Due to the influence of "the power," people feel they must follow and maintain the precedence previously set of fixed ideas, manias, phobias, and prejudices – the established cultural identity. This requires internal dissociation. The individual mind blocks out the humanity of a sacrificial victim and transforms the victim into an object.

Suggestion is reinforced by:

1) **Repetition**
2) **Duration of facts**
3) **Prestige of the idea**

Those more open to suggestion are the young, women, people who identify with a culture, and the criminology inclined.

Suggestion may lead to a *Shared Psychotic Disorder* and a *Culture-Bound Syndrome*.

Genital Blood Ritual Suggestion

Arguments promoting Genital Blood Ritual are subtle, hidden, and protected by claims of religious demand or professional expertise.

Because religious and medical false rationalizations for the ritual cannot withstand genuine, unbiased, objective inquiry, the impetus behind the ritual required hard-hitting emotional appeals that bypass the rational intellect. **The God Excuse**.

Marking the body and cutting the genitals have evolved from pagan rituals and signs of tribal identification. Tribal body-marking practices evolved into primitive religious rituals, a form of worshipping the dead, and eventually adopted into the vaster secular scientific, medical format.

In primitive tribes, the group trumps the individual, ritual trumps individualism. Ritual makes all tribe members subservient to the social norm and culture of conformity. Tribal programming structures and compartmentalizes thought. This makes an "us vs them" mentality.

> **History fades into fable; fact becomes clouded with doubt and controversy; the statue falls from the pedestal. Columns, arches, pyramids, what are they but heaps of sand; and their epitaphs, but characters written in the dust,**
> *Washington Irving.*

Medical

The most noble part of the art of medicine
Is knowing when to do nothing

Dr. Ignatz Semmelweis, prior to Pasteur, recommended that before seeing patients, as during child birth, doctors should wash their hands after an autopsy. He was ridiculed and his right to practice medicine was taken from him.

> **SEMMELWEIS REFLEX**: The Semmelweis Reflex is the dismissal or rejecting out of hand any formulation, automatically, without thought, inspection, or experiment

Cloaked Authority

Genital alterations of minors are performed on healthy patients and is therefore beyond a treatment of physical disease. Consequently, through the combined Cloak of Authority of the medical smock and/or clerical robe, they have become socialized medico-religious ritual experts replacing parental authority, and for some, even their own religious authority. Dr. Catherine Bell in *Ritual Theory, Ritual Practice* wrote:[130]

> As institutions of specialists take on the formulation of reality, there is a decreased need for personal or collective rituals to assume that function. Ultimately, when the strategies of ritualization are dominated by a specific group, recognized as official experts, the definition of reality that they objectify works primarily to retain the status and authority of the experts themselves.

Specific relations of domination and subordination are generated and orchestrated by the participants themselves simply by participating.

It is this type of control that must be understood. These bodies of knowledge act simultaneously to secure a particular form of authority.

Sexuality The Feminine Travail

Women are not the leisured sex.

Just as prepuce restoration where the remaining penile skin must be stretched, doctors use the stretching technique with females who are born without a vagina, a condition termed Congenital Vaginal Aplasia to create a vagina. And, there are many other female developmental conditions.

These is more likely than not the reason for all the different virgin priestess and servant sects dotting the landscape of human religions.

Though the priestesses were to be virgins made a good concept for those with no vagina. Yet, it did not eliminate anal sex where they could reach orgasm from the anal g-spot.

There are women who prefer anal sex due the fact it has been researched the women achieve a stronger and higher instance of orgasm.

Congenital Anomalies → Vulva and Vagina

From the Mayo Clinic web site:

Vaginal agenesis (a-JEN-uh-sis) is a rare disorder in which the vagina doesn't develop, and the womb (uterus) may only develop partially or not at all.

These conditions are present before birth and may also be associated with kidney or skeletal problems. Vaginal agenesis is often identified at puberty when a female does not begin menstruating. **If she has not had a menstrual period by age 15, it is time to see a doctor**.

The condition is also known as mullerian agenesis, mullerian aplasia, or Mayer-Rokitansky-Kuster-Hauser Syndrome.

Vaginal dilators are used to help aid the problem by stretching the rudimentary skin area where the vaginal opening should be. The instrument is tubular, starting with the size of a pencil, that can used and upgraded in size over a period of time is often successful in creating a vagina.

In some cases, surgery may be needed to make it possible to have vaginal intercourse.

This is similar to those men who are now stretching their penile skin to recreate a penile prepuce that takes years to achieve.

Signs and Symptoms

As vaginal agenesis often goes unnoticed until females reach their teens, but don't menstruate (amenorrhea), other signs of puberty usually follow typical female development.

Vaginal agenesis may have these features:

1) The external genitals look like a typical female
2) The vagina may be shortened without a cervix at the end, or absent and marked only by a slight indentation where the vaginal opening would typically be located.

3) There may be no uterus or one that is only partially developed. If there is tissue lining the uterus (endometrium), monthly cramping or chronic abdominal pain may occur.
4) The ovaries are typically fully developed and functional, but may be in an unusual location in the abdomen. Sometimes the pair of the fallopian tubes that eggs travel through to get from the ovaries to the uterus are absent or do not develop typically.

Vaginal agenesis may also be associated with:

1) Problems with development of the kidneys and urinary tract.
2) Developmental changes in the bones of the spine, ribs and wrists.
3) Hearing problems.
4) Other congenital conditions that also involve the heart, gastrointestinal tract and limbs.

Causes

It is not clear what causes vaginal agenesis, but at some point, during the first 20 weeks of pregnancy, tubes called the mullerian ducts do not develop properly.

The Mullerian duct is the embryonic structure that develops into the female reproductive tract including the oviduct, uterus, cervix and upper vagina. This structure is essential mammalian function in providing the site of fertilization, embryo implantation and fetal development.

Typically, the lower portion of these ducts develops into the uterus and vagina, and the upper portion becomes the fallopian tubes. Underdevelopment of the mullerian ducts results in an absent or partially closed vagina, absent or partial uterus, or both.

Complications

Vaginal agenesis may impact sexual function, but after treatment the reconstructed vagina will function well for sexual intercourse.

Females with a missing or partially developed uterus cannot get pregnant. Yet, if the ovaries are healthy, it may be possible to have a baby through in vitro fertilization. The embryo can be implanted in the uterus of another female to carry the pregnancy.

Research

Genetic Psychology and Evolutionary Psychology are fairly new Disciplines with their corresponding Journals. Research is expanding knowledge in these fairly new areas of study.

People must be careful interpreting behavior to a single line of genetics within people. Much negative behavior exudes from severe child abuse as occurred to Hitler and Stalin as well as consequences of circumcision with a minimum of more 1 in 7 complication rate.

Medico/Religious Psychopathic Impairment

Lifton in his *The Nazi Doctors* stated sacrifices are Purification Rituals and those participating in this Doubling are living in a self-induced criminal substructure:

> The Nazi doctor knew that he selected, but did not interpret selections as **murder**. One level of disavowal, then, was the Auschwitz self's altering of the **meaning of murder**; and on the other, the repudiation by the original self of anything done by the Auschwitz self.

Indeed, disavowal was the life blood of the Auschwitz self... Doubling can include elements considered characteristic of **psychopathic character impairment;** *... Doubling may well be an important psychological mechanism for individuals living within any* **criminal substructure.**

They think they are doing constructive work in a slaughterhouse.

And my rule is: You break it, you bought it.
Yaz. *Double Team.*

Legal

Cultural Convention Usurps the Rule of Law

In 1996 a bill making Female Genital Mutilation (FGM) of minors a crime was passed.[131] Yet infant and child cliteroidectomy, cliteroplasty and labioplasty on children continues. In addition, male minors are not protected by the FGM law though Section 1 of the 14th Amendment states:[132]

> *All persons born or naturalized in the United States, and subject to the jurisdiction thereof, are citizens of the United States and of the United States and of the States wherein they reside. No State shall make or enforce any law which shall abridge the privileges or immunities of citizens of the United States; nor shall any State deprive any person of life, or property, without due process of law; nor deny to any person within its jurisdiction the equal protection of the laws.*

The FGM bill deprives the male child of equal rights, the right to privacy and due process. According to the existing law, protection of the male cannot extend from the FGM bill; a separate bill is required.

Now since the Muslim court decision a new bill for all children is required or overturn the Detroit court decision.

Deliberate Indifference and Deliberate Difference

Deliberate Indifference originated from prison inmate suits detailing a lack of, denial of, or delay in needed medical care.[133] The opposite of Deliberate Indifference is Deliberate Difference.

120

There is either: **1):** special consideration given an individual or group of persons; or, **2):** overt and unnecessary action which harms one person or group of persons while those outside that group are protected from harm.

DELIBERATE DIFFERENCE: setting apart an individual or identifiable group, either expressly or by mute sanction, for different laws, equality, equity, actions, or inactions.

Socialized Sexual Harassment

Sexual harassment is improper conduct of a sexual nature, including: verbal, physical, and visual conduct that is unsolicited and unwelcome.

Title VII of the 1964 Civil Rights Act is the law used for most sexual harassment claims.

To file a sexual harassment claim one does not need to be the person harassed. All that is necessary is to show a hostile environment exists or a quid pro quo has occurred. An institution is liable whether it knew, aided, or did not know sexual harassment occurred.   It is the institution's responsibility to protect.

Genital rituals constitute a socially sanctioned form of Socialized Sexual Harassment. There are two types of crime that are used by sexual harassment actions: *hostile environment*, and *quid pro quo*.

Hostile Environment

Hostile Environment's sexual harassment, like other sexual crimes, is based on power and dominance.

Dominant attitudes include feeling one is superior, a bias against difference and, required submission, to a perceived selfishly selected altruistic status quo. It is obvious there is a Hostile Environment for Genital Dismemberments regardless of the finery presented.

Quid Pro Quo

Quid Pro Quo comes from the Latin term meaning *this for that*. It implies advantages in return for favors. The point of *quid pro quo*, in the context of this subject matter, is an exchange of something of value for sexual access. Social threats, coercion and extortion are all part of Genital Dismemberment rituals. Whether religious, medical, or tribal, they cost money with someone who charges a fee. Sex is a form of value. The quid pro quo of Genital Dismemberments is a socialized sexual trade-off for whether through religion or the secular.

LEGAL TRIANGLE

Legal basis for settling disputes is a triangle. At the center is *value*.

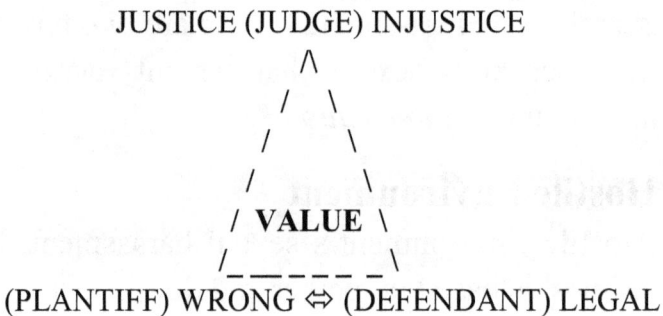

```
          JUSTICE (JUDGE) INJUSTICE
                    /\
                   /  \
                  /    \
                 /      \
                / VALUE  \
               /_ _ _ _ _ _\
(PLANTIFF) WRONG ⇔ (DEFENDANT) LEGAL
```

PROSECUTION

Possible avenues to prosecution, of individuals and health care personnel may possibly be through breaches from, among others, the following:

Agency

An Agent is a representative in a position of great trust and confidence.[134] When it comes to genital alterations of a minor, the doctor's fiduciary relationship is to the child, not the parent or organization. Social Agency responsibility is exclusively to and for the child.

An Agent's power, control, and authority are supposed to be of a supportive capacity, yet in performing a Genital Blood Ritual, or procedure, a person who alters genitals is not neutral because they also derive benefit – monetary gain, social standing, or both.

So, we see that the pressure exerted in favor of the procedure may be due to something other than potential benefit of the child.

Assault and Battery

Given that genital injury is non-Jerusalemic, it is unlawful in religious origin, and it is not immune from civil protection when claimed to be medicine.

ASSAULT is a general intent offense requiring only the general *mens rea* (frame of mind) common to any offense. It is a specific intent offense requiring in addition to the general *mens rea* for an assault a special *mens rea*.

AGGRAVATED ASSAULT: an assault where "serious bodily injury" is inflicted on the person assaulted; a particularly fierce or reprehensible assault; an assault exhibiting peculiar depravity or atrocity – including assaults committed with dangerous or deadly weapon; an assault committed with further crime.

BATTERY: "the unlawful application of force to the person of another," the least touching of another person willfully, or in anger, … In tort law the legal protection of battery extends to any part of one's body or to "anything so closely attached thereto that it is customarily regarded as a part thereof."

Assault with Attempt to Disfigure also applies to Genital Alterations.[135]   This occurs often when parent's divorce and one parent alters the child's genitals to punish the other parent[136] This is Specific Intent.[137] Another definition:

ASSAULT is a general intent offense requiring only the general *mens rea* (frame of mind) common to any offense. It is a specific intent offense requiring in addition to the general *mens rea* for an assault a special *mens rea*.

Cause

Cause is the reason and motive for an action. Cause and Effect is the relationship between an action to its result.[138] Cause examines the foreseeability of consequences, and whether or not a person should be held responsible.

CAUSE: that which effects a result. In law "cause" is not a constant and agreed-upon term. The following is a list of some of the attempts to conceptualize "that which effects a result."

DIRECT CAUSE: the active, efficient cause that sets in motion a train of events that brings about a result without the intervention of any other independent source.

IMMEDIATE CAUSE: the nearest cause in point of time and space; it is not necessarily direct or proximate cause.

PROXIMATE CAUSE: that which in natural and continuous sequence unbroken by any new independent cause produces an event, and without which the injury would not have occurred.

REMOTE CAUSE: that which does not necessarily produce an event without which injury would not occur. Thus, a cause which is not considered to be "proximate" will be regarded as "remote."

Coercion

Coercion is the act of compelling by force of authority.[139] It is forced compliance. Coercion changes the nature and range of options in choice. Force may be physical, or mental as: pressure, harassment, threats, or intimidation. In coercion the Con Type of Approach is main in the perpetrator's Modus Operandi.

Cultural Coercion

Cultural Coercion is the fear produced from being forced out of the community. With male circumcision those who disagree will suffer ostracism. In many parts of Africa, Judaism and Islam Genital Dismemberment is a requisite to become married. Socially, it in many places dependent of the feminine.

Competence

One is not competent to decide on Genital Dismemberment when lacking knowledge. This may, or may not, be from an institution's purposeful misleading, or omission to reasonably inform. Some people may not be physically or psychologically able to make a proper decision even if facts are presented, though facts are often withheld. Becky Cox White wrote:[140]

> The procedures for Informed Consent include assessing patient's competence... Once patients are determined to be competent, they are given the information and a chance to digest it, ask questions, and relate it to their own value structures.
>
> Patients are competent for the task of giving a free and informed consent if they are generally informable and cognitively capable of making decisions...
>
> The nine individual criteria for competence to consent were assembled under four broad categories: informability, cognitive and affective capability, ability to choose, and ability to recount one's decision-making process.
>
> Informability consists of the capabilities to (1) receive information, (2) recognize relevant information as information, and (3) remember information. Cognitive and affective capability includes the capacities to (4) relate situations to oneself, (5) reason about alternatives, and (6) rank alternatives. Choosing incorporates the abilities to (7) select an option and (8) resign oneself to the choice. Recounting one's decision-making process, alone among the broad capabilities, is not a composite. The only ability here is (9) the only ability here is to explain, by way of recognizable reasons, how one came to one's decision.

This recognition requires that HCP's (Health Care Professionals) (1) provide their patients with full information about the situation in which a choice must be made; (2) work to maximize the patient's ability to understand that information; (3) take care not to coerce patient's choices; and (4) implement autonomous chosen therapies."

Consent

One does not have an obligation to sign an Informed Consent form for a procedure they do not have informed knowledge of. Consent forms given to the parent for Genital Dismemberments and/or Alterations do not include information about the many possible complications. Pozgar wrote, in part:[141]

CONSENT: Simply stated, a voluntary act by which one person agrees to allow someone else to do something.

IGNORANCE OF FACT AND UNINTENTIONAL WRONG: Ignorance of the law is not a defense; otherwise, the ignorant would be rewarded. The fact that a negligent act is unintentional is no defense. Otherwise, defendants could never be found guilty.

FAILURE TO DISCLOSE/INFORMED CONSENT: A physician may be held liable for malpractice if, in rendering treatment to a patient, he or she does not make a proper disclosure to the patient of the risks involved in a procedure… The facts that must be disclosed are those facts the physician knows or should know that a patient needs to be aware of in order to make an informed decision on the course that future medical care will take.

After World War II it became common to Genital Dismember both sexes, without parental consent. Lawsuits have lessened this abuse. Still, there is pressure by hospitals and providers for the procedure.

EXPRESS: To make known explicitly and in declared terms. To set forth an actual *agreement* in words, written or spoken, which unambiguously signifies intent. As distinguished from *IMPLIED* the term is not left to implication or interference from conduct or circumstances. When parties show their *agreement* in words, they create an express *contract* as contrasted to a contract implied by circumstances alone, or a quasi-contract, which is applied in law in order to obtain justice.

Cruel & Unusual Punishment

From anger, hate, envy, and resentments actions of Genital Dismemberments constitute unwarranted punishment whose origins reside in psychosexual power relations.[142] It does not matter if these acts are from the social, medical, religious, or parental.

These violent acts violate the 8th Amendment of the United States Constitution.

Excessive bail shall not be required, nor excessive fines imposed, nor cruel and unusual punishments inflicted.

Duty & Its Breach

Duty[143] is first to the child. Parents, physicians, and other health care professionals, the religious and society are all involved and share responsibility.

DUTY: obligatory conduct owed by a person to another person. In *tort* law, duty is a legally sanctioned obligation the *breach* of which results in the *liability* of the actor. Thus, under the law of *negligence*, if an individual owes to others a DUTY OF CARE, he must conduct himself so as to avoid negligent injury to them.

BREACH OF DUTY: a failure to perform a duty owed to another or to society; a failure exercise that care which a *reasonable man* would exercise under similar circumstances.

BREACH OF PROMISE: failure to do what one promises, where he has promised it in order to induce action in another.

BREACH OF TRUST: violation by a *trustee* of a *duty* which *equity* lays upon him, whether willful and *fraudulent* through *negligence*, or arising through mere oversight or forgetfulness.

BREACH OF TRUST WITH FRAUDLENT INTENT: a larceny after trust, which includes all of the elements of larceny except the unlawful taking in the beginning.

Endangerment, Abandonment & Molestation

Due to the vast number of medical errors, as well as from religious non-clinical procedures, Genital Dismemberments and Alterations constitute Child Endangerment where protection of the minor is abandoned. These rituals, as indeed they are rituals, constitute a form of Socialized Child Molestation.

Extortion and Exaction

Extortion takes something of value by threat of violence or by undue exercise of power anything that is not due them, or more than due them. Extortion creates fear.

Exaction is a forced compliance and obedience as paying dues and fees. Genital Blood Rituals are forms of social dues.

Fraud

Fraud is intentional deception. The burden of "choice" is put upon the parents. But, the 'choice' is a false choice, not a legitimate choice.

Parents of children are pressured by society and medical professionals as well as religious authorities to make a decision between Genital Dismemberments and/or other Alterations. Parents should be protected from the pressures to have their children abused, violated, and have violence put upon them.

With little research, parents will find that under the guise of religious and/or medical necessity, Genital Dismemberments and/or Alterations are not required by their deity or for health or for hygiene. In societies where genitals are not mutilated, there is no social demand for unnaturally altered genitals.

To ease minds, in cases of religious genital blood rituals, people should be informed the Abraham story of his "circumcision covenant" was added by corrupt priests after the return from Babylon in 500BCE.

To eliminate medical and social pressure it should clearly be explained to parents that the child does indeed feel changed and depending will remember the procedure. Not to inform parents of potential problems can be a fraud.

Two basic forms of Fraud are Civil and Criminal. More specifically types of Fraud include, in part: Constructive Fraud, In Factum, Misrepresentation, Wire, Mail and Insurance Fraud. Gaslighting is also a form of Fraud and Abuse. Some are the following:[144]

FRAUD Intentional deception resulting in *injury* onto another. Elements of fraud are: false and material misrepresentation made by one who either knows it is falsity or is ignorant of its truth; the maker's intent that the representation be relied on by the person and in a manner reasonably contemplated; the person's ignorance of the falsity of the representation; the person's rightful or justified reliance; and proximate injury to the person.

CONSTRUCTIVE [LEGAL] FRAUD: Comprises all acts, omissions, and concealments involving breach of equitable or *legal duty*, trust or confidence and resulting in damage to another, no scienter is required. Thus, the party who makes the misrepresentation need not know it is false.

EXTRINSIC [COLLATERAL] FRAUD: Fraud that prevents a party from knowing about his rights or *defenses* or from having a fair opportunity of presenting them at a trial, or from fully *litigating* at the trial all the rights or defenses that he was entitled to.

FRAUD IN FACT [POSITIVE FRAUD]: Actual fraud. Deceit. Concealing something or making a false representation with an evil intent [scienter] when it causes injury to another. It is used in contrast to CONSTRUCTIVE FRAUD (above) which does not require an evil intent.

FRAUD IN LAW: Fraud that is presumed from circumstances, where the one who commits it need not have any evil intent to commit a fraud; it is a *CONSTRUCTIVE FRAUD*.

FRAUD IN THE FACTUM: Generally, arises from a lack of identity or disparity between the *instrument*, executed and the one intended to be executed, or from circumstances which go to the question as to whether the instrument ever had a legal existence; as for example, when a blind or illiterate person executes a deed when it has been read falsely to him after he asked to have it read. Fraud in the factum provides a stronger basis for setting aside an instrument than *FRAUD IN THE INDUCEMENT*.

FRAUD IN THE INDUCEMENT: Fraud which is intended to and which does cause one to execute an *instrument*, or make an agreement, or render a *judgment*. The misrepresentation involved does not mislead one as to the paper he signs but rather misleads as to the true facts of the situation, and the false impression it causes is a basis of a decision to sign or render a judgment.

Hate Crime

Hate Crimes are crimes of intolerance.[145]

A hate crime is a criminal offense committed against persons, property or society that is motivated, in whole or in part, by an offender's bias against an individual or group's race, religion, ethnic/national origin, gender, age disability or sexual orientation.

There are four categories of hate crimes:**1)** Thrill Seeking, **2)** Reactive, **3)** Retaliatory and **4)** Mission.

THRILL exists in ritual events.

1) The offender is motivated by a social or psychological thrill and by the approval of peers

2) Generally, there is no precipitating incident on the part of the victim

3) The offender usually seeks out the victim in the victim's setting

4) The victim is identified as a "different" member of a particular group.

REACTIVE genital mutilation, dismemberments and alterations arise, in part, from being the opposite sex or different religion. Then perpetration stems from the *imago Vivendi*. **(1)** The hate crime is motivated by the perpetrator's perception that an "outsider poses a threat to a way of life." **(2)** Occurrence is chiefly within the perpetrators living space, (Intimidation often turns to physical violence.)

RETALIATION involves **(1)** motivation from prejudice and **(2)** may involve large group activity.

With the **MISSION** type perpetrator: **(1)** All members of the despised group are targeted, **(2)** Offenders believe they are attacking an inferior group, **(3)** Often the perpetrator believes he is instructed by a "higher power." **(4)** There is a sense of urgency; and, **(5)** The perpetrator may suffer from mental illness.

The Mission may be hygienic from fear of penetration giving rise to a purification ritual justified through the *imago Vivendi*. Missions also glorify, be it a glorification of the sex not mutilated being attacked, or the social body in which the inhabitants live.

Intent

Perpetrator intent is not considered in child abuse. To stop social abuses as unwarranted medical and religious genital alterations, defense for the good of the children is inadmissible as a falsity in denial, deferral, deflection, and deceit.[146]

INTENT: a state of mind wherein the person knows and desires the consequences of his act which, for purposes of criminal liability, must exist at the time the offense is committed. The existence of this state of mind is often impossible to prove directly; consequently, it must be determined from reasonable deductions, such as the likelihood that the act in question would result in the consequent injury.

Two general *classes* of intent exist in the criminal law.

GENERAL INTENT, which must exist in all crimes; and,

SPECIFIC INTENT, which is essential to certain crimes and which, must be proved beyond a reasonable doubt.

Mayhem

Mayhem[147] is the taking of a body part, rendering the victim less functional.[148]

MAYHEM: the common law *felony* of maliciously *maiming* or dismembering or in any other way depriving another of the use of any part of his body so as to render him less able to fight in the king's army.

Many States treat *mayhem* as **Aggravated Assault**. Some States retain *mayhem* as a separate offense.

Mens Rea – Frame of Mind

Mens rea is the psychological frame of mind of the person who commits the crime. This is to be considered about the perpetrator who acts, as well as the person who transfers the authority to act.

The following connects: 1) FBI findings regarding sexual homicides, same as Genital Dismemberment actors to, 2) Mens rea.[149],[150]

FRAME OF MIND is a general descriptive term for a dominant emotional state that acts as a primary filter and interpreting mechanism regarding external events. The frame of mind of the offenders just before the crime revealed highly negative emotional states...

These findings suggest that there is little emotion experienced by the killer to interpret the behavior of the victim in the most negative manner. The frame of mind and mood states illustrate how the killer supports his negative cognitions and justification for the crime. There is no emotional reservoir to relate to vulnerability, pain, and fear of the victim.

MENS REA: a guilty mind; the mental state accompanying a forbidden act. For an act to constitute a criminal offense, the act usually must be accompanied by a requisite mental state. Criminal offenses are usually defined within reference to one of four recognized states of mind that accompanies the actor's conduct:

(1): **intentionality**
(2): **knowingly**
(3): **recklessly**
(4): **grossly [criminally] negligent**

Negligence

Negligence is in all phases of Genital Dismemberments.

There is a high incidence of complications in genital alterations.[151] One hundred percent of Genitally Dismembered children will suffer loss of sexual sensation. Willful negligence occurs when information is withheld on purpose, regardless of intent.[152]

NEGLIGENCE: failure to exercise that degree of care which a person of ordinary prudence (a reasonable man [person]) would exercise under the same circumstances. The term refers to conduct which falls below the standard established by law for the protection of others against unreasonable risk of harm.

CONCURRENT NEGLIGENCE: the wrongful acts or omissions of two or more persons acting independently but causing the same injury. The independent actions do not have to occur at the same time, but must produce the same result. The actors are all responsible for paying the damages, and can usually be sued together in one lawsuit or individually in separate lawsuits.

CRIMINAL [CULPABLE] NEGLIGENCE: such negligence as is necessary to incur criminal liability; in most jurisdictions, culpable [criminal] negligence is something more than the slight negligence necessary to support a civil action for damages. Thus, culpable negligence, "under criminal law," is recklessness and carelessness resulting in injury or death, as imports a thoughtless disregard of consequences or a heedless indifference to the safety and rights of others.

WANTON NEGLIGENCE: an intentional act of an unreasonable character in disregard of a risk known, or so obvious that it must have been known, and so great as to make it highly probable that harm would follow. The act is usually accompanied by a conscious indifference to the consequences amounting to willingness that they shall follow. The term "wanton" is used synonymously with WILLFUL, or RECKLESS.

Racketeering

Racketeering is dishonest and fraudulent business dealings. The Rico Act was established in 1970 to combat *racketeering* in organized crime. Section1964C allows civil claims.

Legal provisions appear to apply to Genital Alterations from the actions of some social entities, health care organizations as medical societies, hospitals, and birthing centers; as well as, individuals. Two areas are:

1) **extortion** that involves making an individual willing to give something of value induced through violence, fear (as false health claims about disease consequences if a person is not Dismembered), or under color of official right.

2) the **sexual exploitation** of children under Sections 2251, 2251A, 2252, and 2260 of the Rico Act.

Religious Child Abuse Exemptions

The Native American Ghost Dance, and Vow to the Sun do not apply because they possess Separate Nation Status. The Committee on Bioethics states:

However, the constitutional guarantees of freedom of religion do not sanction harming another person in the practice of one's religion, and do not allow religion to be a legal defense when one harms another... The Committee on Bioethics asserts that: the opportunity to grow and develop safe from physical harm with the protection of our society is the right of every child.

Religious Freedom

The severity of the Jerusalemic Genital Dismemberment increased and in 140 A.D. to full glans exposure away from just the extending tip taken. Jesus had his prepuce without the extending foreskin. Then around 500 A.D. at the time of Mohammad it was altered again with blood sucking of the penis.

Circumcisions of both sexes are NOT part of the three Jerusalemic religions: Judaism, Christianity, or Islam. Therefore, allowing the procedure of circumcision is the United States government creating a new religion regardless of whatever they call themselves.

Congress shall make no laws respecting an establishment of a religion, or prohibiting the free exercise thereof; or abridging the freedom of speech, or of the press, or the right of the people to assemble, and to petition the government for a redress of grievances.

Statute of Limitations

Many States have eliminated time limits in child abuse claims. Recently California has allowed males to sue priests for sexual abuse decades before.

Tort

In creating the social breach by changing the Genital Dismemberment from which religious precedence is claimed with the transference to medicine, both religion and medicine have misguided society's expectations of them.

TORT: a wrong; a private or civil wrong or injury resulting from a breach of legal duty that exists by virtue of society's expectations regarding interpersonal conduct, rather than by contract or other private relationship. The essential elements of a tort are the existence of a legal duty owed by a defendant to a plaintiff, breach of that duty, and a casual relation between defendant conduct and the damage to plaintiff.

Other

Other avenues for prosecution are: solicitation, damages, medical records, and medical staff relationships, because destruction of medical records has occurred during law suits.

If you are neutral in situations of injustice,
You have chosen the side of the oppressor.
Desmond Tutu.

Laws control the lesser man.
Right conduct controls the greater one.
Mark Twain.

CONCLUSION

No aspect of human life seethes with so many un-exorcised demons as does sex. No human activity is so hexed by superstition, so haunted by residual tribal lore, and so harassed by socially induced fear.
Harvey Cox.

Joseph Campbell stated to the effect: **When you participate in a ritual you are participating in a myth**.

Mircea Eliade observed that during a ritual the person/group psychic being transfers to the time/place of the original ritual in which it is based – as with male and female circumcision. This represents **ancestor worship**.

The feminine always comes first. The divine male child comes second. And then, the father comes when the child reaches around puberty. So, it is with the three Jerusalemic religions in patriarchy with their **death cults**.

In the Jungian Mana Family the Mother comes first in the form of Judaism. Second is Christianity's Divine Male Child. And after the Child grows, then enters the Jerusalemic step-Father Islam.

Jung said one is safest in the Child. This bears witness in Jerusalem's Jungian mana family where Genital Dismemberments of both sexes is forbidden and a mortal sin against the feminine Holy Spirit. **It is criminal**.

It's a lot of simple tricks and nonsense.
Han Solo. *Star Wars*.

Bibliography
ANTHROPOLOGY

Bancroft, Anne, *Origins of the Sacred*, Arkana, 1987.

Dawkins, Richard, *The Selfish Gene*, Oxford University Press, 1976.

DeMeo, James, *Saharasia: The 4000 BCE Origins of Child Abuse, Sex-Repression, Warefare and Social Violence, In the Deserts of the Old World*, Natural Energy Works; Illustrated Edition, 2011.

Firestone, Shulamith, *The Dialectic of Sex, The Case for Feminine Revolution*, Bantam, 1979. pp. 1, 2 and 31.

Frazer, James G., *The Belief in Immortality and Worship of the Dead*, Macmillan, New York, NY, 1924.

Hunter, John A and Mannix, Daniel P., *Tales of the African Frontier*, Harper & Brothers, NY, 1954.

Klass, D, & Goss, R., *Dead but not lost: Grief narratives in religious traditions*, AltaMira Press, 1999.

Maccoby, Hyam, *THE SACRED EXACUTIONER: Human Sacrifice and the Legacy of Guilt*, Thames & Hudson, 1983.

Machiavelli, Niccolo, *The Prince*, Written 1613, first published 1532.

Malik, Nadeem, *Corporate Social Responsibility and Development in Pakistan*, Routledge, 2014.

Mbiti, J, *African Religions & Philosophy*. Heinemann, 1990.

Meyers, Carol, *Discovering Eve: Ancient Israelite Women in Context*, Oxford University Press, 1988.

Paine, Thomas, *Common Sense*, Aspen, 1990.

Renfrew, C., & Bahn, P., *Archaeology: Theories, Methods, and Practice*, Thames & Hudson, 2016.

Rousseau, Jean-Jacque, *The Social Contract*, Penguin, 1968.

Ruether, Rosemary Radford, *Sexism and God Talk: Toward a Feminist Theology*, Beacon Press, 1993, p. 107.

BLOOD

Buckley, Thomas and Gottleib, Alma, *Blood Magic: The Anthology of Menstruation*, University of California Press, 1988.

Ehrenreich, Barbara, *Blood Rites: Origins and History of the Passions of War*, Metropolitan, 1997.

Hoffman, Lawrence, *Covenant of Blood: Circumcision and Gender in Rabbinic Judaism*, University of Chicago Press, 1996.X

Horrigan, Bonnie, *Red Moon Passage: The Power and Wisdom of Menopause*, Three Rivers Press, 1996.

Knight, Chris, *BLOOD RELATIONS: Menstruation and the Origin of Culture*, Yale University Press, 1991.

Laferrierer-Rancour, Daniel, *Signs of the Flesh: An Essay on the Evolution of Hominid Sexuality*, Yale University Press, 1991.

Marshall, Paul with Gilbert, Lela, *Their Blood Cries Out*, Word Publishing, 1997.

CRIMINOLOGY

Ambrosio, Giovanna, *On Incest: Psychoanalytic Perspectives*, Routledge, 1988.

DeRiver, Paul J., *The Sexual Criminal: A Psychoanalytical Study*, Charles C. Thomas, 1956.

Douglas, John, Burgess, Ann, Allen and Ressler, Robert, *Crime Classification Manuel: A Standard System for Investigating and Classifying Violent Crimes*, Jossey-Bass, 1997.

Douglas, John with Olshaker, Mark, *Journey into Darkness*, Pocket Books, 1997.

Douglas, John with Olshaker, Mark, *Mind Hunter: Inside the FBI's Elite Serial Crime Unit*, Pocket Books, 1995.

Douglas, John with Olshaker, Mark, *Obsession*, Pocket Books, 1998.

Douglas, John with Olshaker, Mark, *The Anatomy of Motive*, Pocket Books, 1999.

Fairstein, Linda, *Sexual Violence: Our War Against Rape*, Berkeley, 1995.

Fletcher, Connie, *What Cops Know*, Pocket, 1992.

Forward, Susan; Craig Faustus Buck; Craig Buck, *Betrayal of Innocence: Incest and its Devastation*, Penguin Books, 1988.

Goodwin, Jean, *Sexual Abuse: Incest Victims and Their Families*, Year Book Medical Pub., 1989.

Hazelwood, Roy with Michaud, Stephen, *The Evil That Men Do*, St. Martin's True Crime, 2000.

Hazelwood, Robert Roy and Burgess, Ann W., *Practical Aspects of Rape Investigation: A Multi-Disciplined Approach*, Elsevier, 1987.

Holmes, RM and Holmes, *Profiling Violent Crimes: An Investigative Tool*, Sage 2002.

Kelleher, M. and Kelleher, C., *Murder Most Rare: The Female Serial Killer*, Dell, 1998.

Keppel, Robert, *Signature Killers: Interpreting the Calling Cards of Serial Murderers*, Pocket, 1997.

Kincaid, James R., *Erotic Innocence: The Culture of Child Molesting*, Duke University Press, 1998.

Kluft, Richard P., *Incest-Related Syndromes of Adult Psychopathology*, American Psychiatric Publishing, Inc., 1990.

Love, Patricia with Robinson, Jo, *The Emotional Incest Syndrome*, Bantam, 1991.

Maltz, Wendy, *Incest and Sexuality: A Guide to Understanding and Healing,* Lexington Books, 1991.

Monteleone, James A., *Recognition of Child Abuse for the Mandated Reporter*, G W Medical Pub, Inc., 1996.

Ressler, Robert; Burgess, Ann; Douglas, John, *SEXUAL HOMICIDE: Patterns and Motives*, Free Press, 1995.

Ressler, Robert & Shachtman, T., *I Have Lived in the Monster*, St. Martin's, 1997.

Ressler, Robert & Shachtman, T., *Whoever Fights Monsters*, St. Martin's, 1992.

Russell, Diana E. H., *The Secret Trauma: Incest in the Lives of Girls and Women*, Revised Edition, Basic Books, 1987.

Shepher, Joseph, *Incest: A Biosocial View*, Academic Press, 1983.

Spencer, Judith, *Suffer the Child*, Pocket, 1989.

Stephany, Timothy J., *Blood and Incest: The Unholy Beginning of the Universe*, Createspace, 2013.

ETHICS AND MORALITY

Beauchamp T, Childress J, *Principles of Biomedical Ethics*, New York: Oxford University Press, 1979.

Boss, Judith, *Ethics for Life*, McGraw Hill, 2023.

Burnor, Richard; Raley, Yvonne, *Ethical Choices: An Introduction to Moral Philosophy with Cases*, Oxford University Press, 2011.

Finnish, John, *Fundamentals of Ethics*, Georgetown University Press, 1983.

Gillon R., *Philosophical Medical Ethics*, John Wiley and Sons, 1985.

Kamm F.M., *Intricate ethics: Rights, responsibilities, and permissible harm*, Oxford University Press, 2007.

Kreeft, Peter, *Ethics for Beginners: Big Ideas from 32 Great Minds*, Word on Fire, 2024.

Liautaud, Susan, Sweetingham, Lisa, *The Power of Ethics: How to Make Good Choices in a Complicated World*, Simon & Schuster, 2022.

Kidder, Rushworth, *How Good People Make Tough Choices: Resolving the Dilemmas of Ethical Living*, Harper, 2009.

Maxwell, John C., *Ethics 101: What Every Leader Needs to Know*, Center Street, 2005.

Trusted, Jennifer, Moral Principles and Social Values, Routledge, 1995.

Vaughn, Lewis, Pojman, Louis P., *The Moral Life: An Introductory Reader in Ethics and Literature*, Oxford University Press, 2021.

Williams, Bernard, *Morality: An Introduction to Ethics*, HarperCollins, 1972.

FEMALE GENITAL MUTILATION

Alday, Martha W., *Female Genital Mutilation: The Cut that Imprisoned Our Bodies in Pain*, Independently Published, 2022.

Boyle, Elizabeth Heger, *Female Genital Cutting: Cultural Conflict in the Global Community*, Johns Hopkins University Press, 2005.

Burrage, Hilary, *Female Mutilation: The Truth Behind the Horrifying Global Practice of Female Genital Mutilation*, New Holland Publishers, 2016.

Dera, Besma, *Female Genital Mutilation (Salamatu Jalloh story): The Good, The Bad and The Ugly*, Independently Published, 2024.

Dorkenoo, Efua, *Cutting the Rose: Female Genital Mutilation: Female Genital Mutilation: The Practice and Its Prevention*, Minority Rights Publications, 1994.

Heralut, Loraine, *Female Genital Mutilation in France*, Our Knowledge Publishing, 2021.

Hicks, Esther, Hicks, Esther K., *Infibulation: Female Mutilation in Islamic Northeastern Africa*, Routledge, 1996.

Julios, Christina, *Female Genital Mutilation and Social Media*, Routledge, 2020.

Kiminta, Maria; Levin, Tobe, *Kiminta A Maasai's Fight against Female Genital Mutilation*, Uncut/Voices Press, 2015.

Lockhat, Haseena, *Female Genital Mutilation: Treating the Tears*, Libri Publishing, 2004.

Robinett, Patricia, *The Rape of Innocence: female genital mutilation and circumcision in the USA*, Nunzio Press, 2010.

Shalabi, Zouheir, A Woman of Honey, *A Female Genital Mutilation FGM is a crime applied by many Moslems and Africans*, Independently Published, 2020.

Thabet, Hoda, *Female Genital Mutilation in the Middle East: Placing Oman on the Map*, National and University of Iceland, 2018.

Twongyeirwe, Hilda, *Taboo. Voices of Women in Uganda on Female Genital Mutilation*, Uncut/Voices Press, 2015.

LEGAL

Gifis, Steven, *Law Dictionary*, 2nd ed., Baron's Educational Series, 1984.

Johnson, Seigler and Winslade, *Clinical Ethics*, 3rd ed., McGraw Hill, 1984.

Kay, Susan, *The Constitutional Dimensions of an Inmate's Right to Health Care*, National Commission on Health Care by the Corrections and Sentencing Committee, Criminal Justice Section of the American Bar Association, 1991.

Myers, John EB, *Legal Issues in Child Abuse and Neglect Practice*, SAGE Publications, Interpersonal Violence: The Practice Series, 2nd Edition, 1998.

White, Becky, *Competence to Consent*, Georgetown University Press, 1991.

MANIPULATION

Bernays, Edward L., *Crystallization Public Opinion*, Kessinger Publishing, 2004.

Bernays, Edward L., *Propaganda*, Ig publishing, 2002.

Bernays, Edward L., *Public Relations*, Bellmen Publishing Company, 1945.

Bernays, Edward L. and Cutler, Howard, *The Engineering of Consent*, University of Oklahoma Press, 1955.

Burney, Robert, *Codependence: The Dance of Wounded Souls*, Joy to Yor & Me Enterprises, 1995.

Herman, Edward S. and Chomsky, Norm, *Manufacturing Consent: The Political Economy of the Mass Media*, Pantheon, 2002.

Post J., Preston I., and Sachs S., *Redefining the Corporation: Stakeholder Management and Organizational Wealth*, Stanford Business Books, 2002.

Rank, Hugh, *Language and Public Policy*, MacMillan, 1975.

Rank, Hugh, *Pep Talk: How to Analyze Political Language*, Counter-Propaganda Press, 1984.

Rank, Hugh, *Persuasion Analysis: A Companion to Composition*, Counter-Propaganda Press, 1988.

Rank, Hugh, *The Pitch*, Counter-Propaganda Press, 1991.

Seitel, Fraser P., *Practice of Public Relations*, 11th Edition, Prentice Hall, 2010.

MEDICINE

Finkel, Martin, A. and Giardino, Angelo P., *Medical Evaluation of Child Sexual Abuse: A Practical Guide*, Sage, 2001.

LeVay, Simon, *The Sexual Brain*, A Bradford Book, The MIT Press, 1993.

Lifton, Robert J., *THE NAZI DOCTORS: Medical Killing and the Psychology of Genocide*, Basic Books, 2017.

Marlow, DR and Sellew, G., *Textbook of Pediatric Surgery*, W. H. Saunders, 1965.

Marshall, FF, editor, *Urologic Complications, Medical and Surgical, Adult and Pediatric*, Year Book of Medical Pub., 1986.

Mendelsohn, Robert S. *Confessions of a Medical Heretic*, Contemporary Books, 1979.

Mendelsohn, Robert S. *How to Raise a Healthy Child in Spite of Your Doctor*, Ballantine Books, 1987.

Schwartz, WM, Charney, EB, Curry, TA, Ludwig, S, *Pediatric Primary Care: A Problem-Oriented Approach*, 2nd edition, Year Book Medical Publishers, 1990.

MUTILATION

Abu-Sahleih, Dr. Sami Aldeeb, *Male & Female Circumcision: Among Jews, Christians & Muslims*, Shangri-La, 2001.

Abu-Sahleih, Dr. Sami Aldeeb, *To Mutilate in the Name of Jehovah or Allah: Legitimization of Male and Female Circumcision*, Middle East Research Associates, 1994. Original: Ohio State University.

Denniston, George C., Milos, Marilynn Fayre, *Sexual Mutilations: A Human Tragedy*, Plenum Press, 1997.

Klein, Hanny-Lightfoot, *A Woman's Odyssey into Africa, Tracks Across Life*, Nunzio Press, 2009.

Klein, Hanny-Lightfoot, *Children's Genitals Under the Knife: Social Imperatives, Secrecy and Shame*, Nunzio Press, 2009.

Klein, Hanny-Lightfoot, *Prisoners of Ritual: An Odyssey into Female Genital Circumcision in Africa*, Nunzio Press, 2009.

Lewis, J., *In the Name of Humanity*, New York, Eugenics, 1949.

Robinett, Patricia, *The Rape of Innocence: One Woman's Story of Female Genital Mutilation in the U.S.A.*, Nunzio Press, 2010.

MYTHOLOGY

Campbell, Joseph, *The Mythic Image*, Princeton University Press, 1991.

Campbell, Joseph, *The Power of Myth*, Paperback Books, 1988.

Eliade, Mircea, *The Myth of the Eternal Return*, Princeton University Press, 1954.

Eliade, Mircea; trans. Mairet, Philip, *Images and Symbols*, in 'Symbolism of the Centre,' Princeton University Press, 1991, p. 39.

Faulkner, Raymond, trans., (The Papyrus of Ani): *The Egyptian Book of the Dead: The Book of Going Forward by Day*, Chronicle Books, 1981.

Frazier, James George, *The Belief in Immortality and the Worship of the Dead*, Macmillan, 1913.

Garnier, John, *THE WORSHIP OF THE DEAD: Or, the Origin and Nature of Pagan Idolatry and its Bearing Upon the Early History of Egypt and Babylonia*, Franklin Classics, 2018.

Graves, Robert, *The Greek Myths*, Complete Edition, Penguin, 1992.

Graves, Robert and Lindop, Grevel, *The White Goddess*, Farrer, Straus and Giroux, 2nd Edition, 2013.

Honko, Lauri, *NIF Newsletter 4*, Nordic Institute of Folklore, Diatrop Books, 1984.

Murry, Margaret, *The God of the Witches*, Oxford University Press, 1970.

Neumann, Erich, *The Great Mother*, Princeton University Press, 1991.

Sagan, Carl; Elwes, Cary, Narrator, *The Demon-Haunted World: Science as a Candle in the Dark*, Audible Audiobook, Brilliance Audio, 2017.

Slater, Phillip, *The Glory of Hera: Greek Mythology and Greek Family*, Princeton University Press, 1992.

PSYCHOLOGY

Adams, Kenneth, *Silently Seduced: When Parents Make Their Children Partners: Understanding Covert Incest*, HCI, 1991.

American Psychiatric Association, *Diagnostic and Statistical Manual of Mental Disorders, DSN-IV*, 4th edition, American Psychiatric Association, 1996.

Berne, Eric, *Games People Play*, Ballentine, 1964.

deMause, Lloyd, *Foundations of Psychohistory*, Creative Books, 1982.

deMause, Lloyd, *The Emotional Life of Nations*, Other Press, 2002.

deMause, Lloyd, *The History of Childhood: The Untold Story of Child Abuse*, Jason Aronson, 1995.

Dorpat, Theodore L., *Gaslighting, the Double Whammy, Interrogation, and Other Methods of Covert Control in Psychotherapy and Psychoanalysis*, Jason Aronson, 1996.

Edinger, Edward F., *EGO and ARCHETYPE*, Shambhala, 1992.

Edinger, Edward F., *The Mystery of THE CONIUNCTIO Alchemical Image of Individuation*, Inner City Books, 1994.

Estes, Clarissa Pinkola, *Women Who Run with the Wolves: Myths and Stories of the Wild Woman*, Ballentine, 1995.

Favazza, Armando R., *Bodies Under Siege: Self-Mutilation in Culture and Psychiatry*, The Johns Hopkins University Press, 1987.

Freud, Sigmund and Hubback, *Beyond the Pleasure Principle (1922): Human's Struggle Between Eros & Thanatos*, Literary Licensing, LLC, 2014.

Forward, Susan with Buck, Craig, *Toxic Parents: Overcoming their Hurtful Legacy and Reclaiming your Life*, Bantam, 1996.

Forward, Susan with Frazier, Donna, *Emotional Blackmail: When People in Your Life Use Fear, Obligation and Guilt to Manipulate You*, Harper Collins, 1997.

Freud, Sigmund, *Three Essays on the Theory of Sexuality*, Avon Books, 1962.

Freud, Sigmund, *Totem and Taboo*, Dover Publications, 2011.

Harris, Thomas, *I'm OK – You're OK*, Avon Books, 1973.

Hobsbawn, Eric, et al., *The Invention of Tradition: Mass Producing Traditions: Europe, 1970-1914*, Cambridge University Press, 1983.

Holowchak, Andrew; Lavin, Michael, *Repetition: The Compulsion to Repeat, and the Death Drive: An Examination of Freud's Doctrines*, Lexington Books, 2017.

Horney, Karen, *Feminine Psychology*, Norton, 1967.

Jung, Carl Gustav, Ed. Von Franz, Marie-Louise, *Man and his Symbols*, Aldus Books Limited, 1971.

Jung, Carl Gustav, *Psychology of the Unconscious*, Dover Publications, 2012.

Jung, Carl Gustav, *The Archetypes and the Collective Unconscious*, Princeton University Press, 1981.

Jung, Carl Gustav, *The Undiscovered Self*, A Mentor Book, 1958.

Jung, Emma, *ANIMUS and ANIMA*, Spring Publications, 1957.

Little, Margaret, *Transference Neurosis & Transference Psychosis*, Jason Aronson, 1993.

Maslow, Abraham, *Toward A Psychology of Being*, Start Publishing, 2013.

Miller, Alice, *Banished Knowledge: Facing Childhood Injuries*, Anchor, 1991.

Miller, Alice, *Breaking Down the Walls of Silence*, Doubleday, 1990.

Miller, Alice, *For Your Own Good: Hidden Cruelty in Child-rearing and the Roots of Violence*, The Noonday Press, 1990.

Miller, Alice, *The Untouched: Tracing Childhood Trauma in Creativity and Destructiveness*, Anchor. 1991.

Miller, Alice, *Thou Shalt Not Be Aware: Society's Betrayal of the Child*, Farrar, Straus and Giroux, 1998.

Rutter, Virginia, *Woman Changing Woman*, Harper San Francisco, 1993.

Stern, Robin, *The Gaslight Effect: How to Spot and Survive the Hidden Manipulation Others Use to Control Your Life*, Random House, 2007.

Thomas, WI, *Sex and Society: Studies in the Social Psychology of Sex*, University of Chicago Press, 1907.

Vankin, Shmeul (Sam), *Malignant Self-Love: Narcissism Revisited*, Narcissist Publications, 2007.

RITUAL

Bell, Catherine, *Ritual Theory Ritual Practice*, Oxford University Press, 1992.

Heesterman, F. C., *The Inner Conflict of Tradition*, University of Chicago Press, 1985.

Hobbsbawn, Eric, et al., *The Invention of Tradition*. University of Chicago Press, 1982.

Myss, Caroline, *Sacred Contracts: Awakening Your Divine Potential*, Three Rivers Press, 2003.

Rappaport, Roy, and Hurt, Keith, *Ritual and Religion in the Making of Humanity*, Cambridge University Press, 1982.

SCRIPTURAL

Farah, Caesar, *Islam*, Baron's Educational Series, 1994.

Williams, John Alden, *The Word of Islam*, University of Texas Press, 1994.

PERIODICALS

ABUSE

Asher, Richard. "Munchausen Syndrome," *Lancet*, i: 33-41.

Belinksy, J., "Child Maltreatment: An ecological integration," *American Psycholo*, 35, (40: 320-35).

Bools C, Neale BA, "Co-morbidity Associated with Fabricated Illness (Munchausen Syndrome by Proxy)," *Archives of Diseases in Childhood*, 67: 77-79.

Bools C, Neale BA, and Meadow R, "Munchausen syndrome by proxy: a study of psychopathology," *Child Abuse and Neglect*, vol. 18, no 9, pp. 773-88.

Boros, SJ, Ophoven JP, et al., "Munchausen syndrome by proxy: a profile of medical child abuse," *Australian Family Physician*, vol. 24, no. 5, pp. 722-3; 768-69.

Crouse, KA, (1992). "Munchausen Syndrome by Proxy: Recognizing the Victim," *Pediatric Nursing*, 18(3): 249-52.

deMause, L., "The Universality of Incest," *The Journal of Psychohistory*, Fall 1991, Vol.19, No 2, 123-61.

deMause, L., updated, "The Universality of Incest," *The Journal of Psychohistory*, 21, (4), 1994.

Gould, C, "Denying Ritual Abuse of Children," *The Journal of Psychohistory*, 22 (3) 1995.

Meadow, Roy, (1977). "Munchausen Syndrome by Proxy: The Hinterland of Child Abuse," *Lancet*, ii: 342-345.

Menage, J, "Professionals should not collude with abusive systems," *BMJ*, 311:1088-1089, 21 October 1995.

Mire, S, "Genital Mutilation by Any Other Name," *NOCIRC*, Fall, vol.7, No2, p. 1.

Summit, Rowland, "The Child Sexual Abuse Accommodation Syndrome," *Child Abuse and Neglect*, 7: 1777, 1983.

Watson, JL, Rawski, ES, *Death Ritual in Late Imperial and Modern China*, University of California Press, 1998.

CRIMINOLOGY

Babazadeh, Natasha, "Concealing Evidence: 'Parallel Construction,' Federal Investigations, and the Constitution," *Virginia Journal of Law &Technology*, University of Virginia, Fall 2018, Vol.22, No. 01

Bromberg W, and Coyle E, "Rape: A Compulsion to Destroy," Medical Insight, 1974, April, 21-22, 24-25.

Dietrich D, BerkowitzI, Kadushin A, McGloin J, (1990) "Some factors influencing abusers' justification of their child abuse," *Child Abuse and Neglect*, 14, 337-345.

Geberth VJ, "Psychological Profiling," *Law and Order*, 1981, pp. 46-49.

Hartman CR, Burgess AW, "The Genetic Roots of Child Sexual Abuse." *J of Psychotherapy and the Family*, 1986, 2 (2), 83-92.

Hazelwood, Robert R., "The Criminal Sexual Sadist," *Law Enforcement Bulletin*, (FBI), February 1992.

Lanning, Kenneth V., "Child Molesters: A Behavioral Analysis," *National Organization for Missing and Exploited Children*, 1992.

MacCollough MJ, Snowden PR, Wood PJW, Mills HE, "Sadistic Fantasy: Sadistic Behaviors and Offending," *British Journal of Psychiatry*, 1983, 143: 20-29.

Mendelsohn, B, "The Origin of the Doctrine of Victimology," *Excerpta Criminologica*, 1963, 3:239-44.

Podilsky, E, "Sexual Violence," *Medical Digest*, 1996, 34:60-63.

Ressler, Robert K., Burgess, Ann W., "Crime Scene and Profile Characteristics of Organized and Disorganized Murderers," *FBI Law Enforcement Bulletin*, vol. 54, No. 8, August1985, pp. 18-25.

Roth S, Lebowitz L, "The Experience of Sexual Trauma," *Journal of Traumatic Stress*, 1988, Vol1:79-107.

ETHICS AND MORALITY

Avlaro, Carlo, "Ethical Subjectivism: A Lost Cause," Filosofija Sociologija, t.34, Nr3, 2023, pp. 234-243.

Baumeister R.F., Bratslavsky E., Finkenauer C., Vohs K.D. "Bad is stronger than good." *Review of General Psychology*. 2001;5(4):323–370.

Bering, JM, "Intuitive conceptions of dead agents' minds: The natural foundations of afterlife beliefs as phenomenological boundary," *Journal of Cognition and Culture*, 2:263-308, 2002.

Black, D., "In deference of situational ethics, the NHS and permissive society," *J. Med Ethics*, 10(3): 121, Sept 1984.

Card, Dallas; Smith, Noah A., "On Consequentialism and Fairness," *Frontiers in Artificial Intelligence*, 3: 34, 2020.

Dungan J., Waytz A., Young L. "Corruption in the context of moral trade-offs." *Journal of Interdisciplinary Economics*. 2014;26(1-2):97–118.

Editor, "Ethical Drift: Values vs. Standards,' *Ethical Issues in Nursing*, November 8, 2010. Cited from: Kleinman, C.S. (2006) Ethical drift: when good people do bad things." *JONA's Healthcare Law: Ethics and Regulation*, 8(3), 72-76.

Everett, Jim AC; Faber, Nadira S; Savulescu, Julian; Crockett, Molly J, "The costs of being consequentialist: Social inference from instrumental harm and impartial beneficence," *J Exp Soc Psychol*, 2018, Nov; 79: 200-216.

Franz, D.J., "Is Applied Ethics Morally Problematic?" *J Acad Ethics* 20, 359–374 (2022).

Garcia, AG; Green, W, "Subjectivism and the Framework of Constitutive Grounds," *Ethic Theory Moral Pract*, 21, 155-167, (2018).

Goodwin, P.; Darley JM, "The psychology of meta-ethics: Exploring objectivism," *Cognition*, Volume 106, Issue 3, March2008, pp. 1339-1366.

Iaccarino, Maurizio, "Science and Ethics," *National Library of Medicine*, 15 September 2001.

Jablonski, Donald, "When doctors "drift," questions of competency and ethics are key," *Newsletter, North Carolina Medical Board*, Aug 03, 2010.

Kahane G., Everett J.A.C., Earp B.D., Caviola L., Faber N.S., Crockett M.J., Savulescu J. "Beyond sacrificial harm: A two-dimensional model of utilitarian psychology." *Psychological Review.* 2018;125(2):131–164.

Kahane G., Everett J.A.C., Earp B.D., Farias M., Savulescu J. "'Utilitarian' judgments in sacrificial moral dilemmas do not reflect impartial concern for the greater good." *Cognition.* 2015;134:193–209.

Kleinman, Carole S., "Ethical Drift: when good people do bad things," *JONAS Healthc Law Ethics Regul*, 2006, July-Sept;8(3):72-6.

Megías, A.; de Sousa, L; & Jiménez-Sánchez, F., "Deontological and Consequentialist Ethics and Attitudes Towards Corruption: A Survey Data Analysis," *Soc Indic Res* 170, 507–541 (2023). {Deontological = Duty-Based Ethics}

Misselbrook, Davit, "Virtue Ethics – an old answer to a new dilemma? Part 1. Problems with contemporary medical ethics." *J. R. Soc Med*, 2015 Feb, 108(2): 53-56.

Moore, Asher, Emotivism: Theory and Practice," *Journal of Philosophy*, Vol. 55, No. 9, (April 24, 1958), pp. 375-382.

Pitak-Arnnop, Porfamate; Dhanuthai, Kittipong; Hemprich, Alexander; Pausch, Niels C., "Morality, ethics, norms and research misconduct," *J Conserv Dent*, 2012 Jan-Mar; 15(1): 92-93.

Pratt, Cornelius B., "Critique of the classical theory of situational ethics," *Public Relations Review*, Volume 19, Issue 3, Autumn 1993, pp. 219-234.

Quintelier, Katinka; Van Speybroeck, Linda, Braeckerman, Johan, "Normative Ethics Does Not Need a Foundation: It Needs More Science," *Acta Biotheor*, 2011; 59(1): 29-51.

Sternberg, RJ, "Ethical Drift," *Association of American Colleges & Universities*, Summer 2012, Vol.98, No. 3.

Tenbrunsel, Ann E.; Messick, David M., "Ethical Fading: The Role of Self-Deception in Unethical Behavior," Social Justice Research, January 2004, 17(2):223-236.

Tillman, C. Justice; Gonzales, Katerina; Whitman, Marilyn V.; Crawford, Wayne C.; Hood, Anthony C., "A Multi-Functional View of Moral Disengagement: Exploring the Effects of Learning the Consequences," *Front Psychol*, 2017; 8: 2286.

Graves, Robert, *The Greek Myths*, Complete Edition, Penguin, 1992.

FEMALE GENITAL MUTILATION

Abdel-Azim S., "Psychosocial and sexual aspect of female circumcision," *Afr J Urol*. 2013;19:141–2.

Afifi M., "Women's empowerment and the intention to continue the practice of female genital cutting in Egypt," *Archives of Iranian Medicine*. 2009;12(2).

Ahmadi AB., "An analytical approach to female genital mutilation in West Africa," *Int J Women's Res*. 2013;3:37–56.

Al-Hussaini TK., "Female genital cutting: types, motives and perineal damage in laboring Egyptian women," *Med Princ Pract*. 2003;12(2):123–8.

Alsibiani SA, Rouzi AA, "Sexual Function in Women with Female Genital Mutilation," *Fertil Steril*. 2010;93(3):722–4.

Asekun-Olarinmoye E., Amusan O., "The impact of health education on attitudes towards female genital mutilation (FGM) in a rural Nigerian community," *European Journal of Contraception and Reproductive Health Care.* 2008;13(3):289–297.

Awusi VO., "Tradition vs. female circumcision; a study of female circumcision among the Isoko tribe of Delta state of Nigeria," *Bien J Postgrad Med.* 2009;11:1–9.

Ayotunde T, Martin EP, Oludare OA, "Female genital mutilation/cutting in Nigeria: Any abandonment yet?" *Ife Soc Sci Rev.* 2015;24:2.

Babalola S., Brasington A., Agbasimal A., "Impact of a communication programme on female genital cutting in eastern Nigeria," *Tropical Medicine and International Health.* 2006;11(10):1594–1603.

Berer M., "The history and role of the criminal law in anti-FGM campaigns: Is the criminal law what is needed, at least in countries like Great Britain?" *Reproductive Health Matters.* 2015;23(46):145–157.

Berg RC, Denison E, "Effectiveness of interventions designed to prevent female genital mutilation/cutting: a systematic review," *Stud Fam Plann*, 2012;43(2):135–46.

Berg RC, Underland V, Odgaard-Jensen J, Fretheim A, Vist GE, "Effects of female genital cutting on physical health outcomes: A systematic review and meta-analysis," *BMJ Open.* 2014;4:e006316.

Bjork, Malin, "Female genital mutilation is a way to control women's bodies and sexuality," *Topics: European Parliament*, 2017.

Black J, "Female genital mutilation in Britain," *BMJ*, 1995:310:1590-92.

Boyle E., Corl A., "Law and culture in a global context: Interventions to eradicate female genital cutting," *Annual Review of Law and Social Sciences.* 2010;6:195–215.

Broussard P., "The importation of female genital mutilation to the West: The cruelest cut of all," *University of San Francisco Law Review.* 2009;44:787.

Bunei E., Rono J., "A critical understanding of resistance to criminalization of female genital mutilation in Kenya," *Palgrave Handbook of Criminology and the Global South.* 2018:901–912.

Costello S., Quinn M., Tatchell A., "A tradition in transition: Female genital mutilation/cutting; A literature review, an overview of prevention programs and demographic data for Victoria, Australia," *Family Planning Victoria.* 2014.

Diop N., Askew I., "The effectiveness of a community-based education program on abandoning female genital mutilation cutting in Senegal," *Study in Family Planning.* 2009;40(4):307–318.

Dirie MA, Lindmark G, "The risk of medical complications after female circumcision." *East African Med J, 1992: 69(9): 479-482.*

Dunn F., "Is it possible to end female circumcision in Africa?" *Clinical Journal of Obstetric Gynecology.* 2018;1:7–13.

Fernandez-Aguilar S, Noel J-C, "Neuroma of the of the clitoris after female genital cutting," *Obstet Gynecol,* 2003:101:1053-4.

Ghadially, R., 'All for "Izzat": "The practice of female circumcision among Bohra Muslims", *Manushi,* no. 66, September–October 1991.

Grisaru N et al., "Ritual Female Genital Surgery among Ethiopian Jews," *Archives of Social Behavior,* 1997, 26 (20): 1997.

Hamid R., "Female genital mutilation: A tragedy for women's reproductive health," *Afr J Urol.* 2013;19:130–3.

Jones, W.K., et al., "Female Genital Mutilation. Female Circumcision. Who is at Risk in the U.S.?" *Public Health Reports,* 112, no. 5 (1997): 368–77.

Kafatos, F., "Changing culture to end FGM," Lancet, 2018;391(10119):401.

Kouba, L. and Muasher J. "Female Circumcision in Africa: An Overview." *African Studies Review*, 28:95-119.

Larsen U, Okonofua FE. "Female circumcision and obstetric complications," *Int J Gynaecol Obstet*. 2002;77:255–65.

Livermore L, Monteiro R, Rymer J., "Attitudes and awareness of female genital mutilation: A questionnaire-based study in a Kenyan hospital," *J Obstet Gynaecol*. 2007;27:816–8.

Magoha GA, Magoha OB. "Current global status of female genital mutilation: A review," *East Afr Med J*. 2000;77:268–72.

Mahmoud HI, "Effect of female genital mutilation on female sexual function," Alexandria, Egypt, *Alex J Med*. 2016;5:55–9.

Mohamud M., Kaba M., Tamire M., "Assessment of barriers of behavioral change to stop FGM practice among women of Kebri Beyah district, Somali regional state, eastern Ethiopia," *Global Journal of Medical Research*. 2017.

McDonald CF, "Circumcision of the Female," *GP*, 1958; XVIII (3):98-99.

McGee S., "Female circumcisers in Africa: Procedures, rationales, solutions and the road to recovery," *Wash Lee Race Ethnic Anc LJ*. 2005 11:133.

Meniru GI, Meniru MO, Ezh UO, "Female Genital Mutilation," *BMJ*, 1995:311:1088 (21 October).

Montague A. "Infibulation and Defibulation in the Old and New Worlds," *Am Anthropologist*, 47: 464-467, 1945.

Mpinga EK, Macias A, Hasselgard-Rowe J, Kandala NB, Félicien TK, Verloo H, et al., "Female genital mutilation: A systematic review of research on its economic and social impacts across four decades," *Glob Health Action.* 2016;9:31489.

Muteshi, Jacinta K.; Miller, Suellan; Belizan, Jose M., "The ongoing violence against women: Female Genital Mutilation/Cutting," *Reproductive Health*, 13: no. 44, 2016.

Nolen, Stephanie, "Female Genital Cutting Continues to Increase Worldwide," *New York Times*, March 7, 2024.

Ofor MO, Ofor NM, "Female genital mutilation; the place of culture and the debilitating effects on the dignity of the female gender," *Eur Sci J.* 2015;11:14.

Ogbu AC. "Female genital mutilation in Nigeria; a brief sociological review," *World J Prev Med.* 2018;6:1–5.

Okeke T, Anyaehie U, Ezenyeaku C., "An overview of female genital mutilation in Nigeria," *Ann Med Health Sci Res.* 2012;2:70–3.

Olalekan, OA; Ilupej, NA, "Female Genital Mutilation; culture, religion, and medicalization, where do we direct our searchlights for it education: Nigeria as a Case Study," *Tzu Chi Med J*, 2019, Jan-Mar; 31(1): 1-4.

Picters G, Lowenfels AB, "Infibulation in the Horn of Africa." *New York State J of Med*, Vol. 77, No. 6, pp.729-31, April 1977.

Quanta, Ahmed, "And Now: Female Genital Mutilation Comes to America," *Daily Beast*, May 5, 2017.

Rashid AK, Patil SS, Valimalar AS, "The Practice of Female Genital Mutilation among the Rural Malays in North Malaysia." *The Internet Journal of Third World Medicine*, 2010;9(1):1–8.

Romero, Talia Jiminez, "Is Female Genital Mutilation (FGM) on the rise in Europe," *European Society of Religion and Society*, (EARS), 2024.

Saadye, Ali; de Viggiani, Nick; Abzhaparova, Aida; Salmon, Debra; Gray, Selena, "Exploring young people's interpretations of female genital mutilation in the UK using a community-based participatory research approach," *BMC Public Health*, 20 July, 2020.

Serourx, G. I., "Medicalization of female genital mutilation/cutting," *African Journal of Urology*, Volume 19, Issue 3, September 2013, Pages 145-149.

Shah P., "Cutting female genital mutilation from the United States: A European-influenced proposal to alter state and federal legal responses when affording relief to Somali victims in Minnesota," *Cardozo Journal of Law and Gender*. 2015;22:583.

Sharfi AR, Elmegboul MA, Abdella AA, "The continuing challenge of female genital mutilation in Sudan," *Afr J Urol*. 2013;9:136–40.

Shell-Duncan, Bettina, "The medicalization of female 'circumcision': harm reduction or promotion of a dangerous practice," *Social Science & Medicine*, Volume 52, Issue 7, April 2001, Pages 1013-1028.

Shell-Duncan B., Sherlund Y., "Are there 'stages of change' in the practice of female genital cutting?: Qualitative research findings from Senegal and The Gambia" *Afr J Reprod Health*, 2006;10(2):57–71.

Shell-Duncan B., Wander K., Hernlund Y., Moreau A., "Legislating change? Responses to criminalizing female genital cutting in Senegal," *Reproductive Health, Law and Society Review,* 2017;2013;1447(1)(4):63. 803–835.

Turner D., "Female genital cutting: implications for nurses," *Nurs Women's Health*, 2007;11(4):366–72.

Varol N., Turkmani S., Black K., "The role of men in abandonment of female genital mutilation: A systematic review," *BMC Public Health*. 2015;15(1):1034.

Waigwa S., Doos L., Bradbury-Jones C., Taylor J., "Effectiveness of health education as an intervention designed to prevent female genital mutilation/cutting (FG-M/C): A systematic review," *Reproductive Health.* 2018;15(1):62.

Williams-Breault, Beth D, "Eradicating Female Genital Mutilation/Cutting: Human Rights-Based Approaches of Legislation, Education, and Community Empowerment," *Health Hum Rights*, 2018, Dec; 20(2): 223-233.

Wuest S, Raio L, Wyssmueller D, Mueller MD, Stadlmayr W, Surbek DV, et al., "Effects of female genital mutilation on birth outcomes in Switzerland," *BJOG.* 2009;116:1204–9.

LEGAL

Brownies, Sharon, "In the Name of Ritual: An Unprecedented Legal Case focuses on Genital Politics," *U.S. News and World Report.*

Brigman WF, "Circumcision as Child Abuse: The Legal and Constitutional Issues," *Journal of Family Law*, vol. 23, no. 3, 1984-5, pp. 337-357.

Chessler A, "Justifying the Unjustifiable: Rite V. Wrong," 45, *Buffalo Law Rev*, 555, (1997).

Denniston GC, "Circumcision and the Code of Ethics," *Humane Health Care International*, April, 1996, 12.

Denniston GC, "Circumcision Violates All Seven Principles of Medical Ethics," 82, *Cal Law Rev*, 1371, (1994).

Dwyer JG, "Parents' Religion and Children's Welfare: Debunking the Doctrine of Parents' Rights," 82, *Cal Law Rev*, 1371, (1994).

Dwyer GJ, "The Children We Abandon: Religious exemptions to child welfare and education laws as denials of equal protection to children of religious objectors," 74, *North Carolina Law Review*, 1321-1478, (June 1996).

Garrison MR, "Child Sexual Abuse Accommodation Syndrome: Issues of Admissibility in Criminal Trials," *IPT Journal*, vol. 10, 1998.

Holder A, "Law & medicine: circumcision," *JAMA*, vol. 218, no. 1. (Oct. 4, 1971): 149-50.

Mason C, "Exorcising Excision: medico-legal Issues Arising from Male and Female Genital Surgery to Australia," *Journal of Law and Medicine*, (Australia), Vol 9, No. 1: pp. 58-67, August 2001.

Miller, Geoffrey, "Circumcision: Cultural-legal Analysis," *Virginia J of Social Policy & the Law*, Vol. 9: 497-585, Spring 2002.

Morse H, "Law and medicine: ritual circumcision," *JAMA*, vol. 203, no. 12 (March 18,1968): 257-8.

Povenmire R., "Do Parents have the Legal authority to consent to the surgical Amputation of Normal Healthy Tissue from Their Infant children: The Practice of Circumcision in the United States?" 7. *J of Gender, Social Policy & Law*, 87 (1998-1999).

U.S. Department of Justice, "Dignity Health Agrees to Pay $37 Million to Settle False Claims Act Allegations," *Office of Public Affairs*, Oct. 30, 2014.

Van Howe R, Svoboda JS, "Involuntary circumcision: the legal issues, *BJU International*, 1999, 83, Supplement, 1: 63-73.

Wu, Tim, "Is the First Amendment Obsolete," *Columbia Public Law,* Research Paper, No., 14-573.

Zitter J, "Liability for Medical Malpractice in Connection with Performance of Circumcision," *American Law Reports*, 4, 710, (1975).

MEDICAL

Dawson B, "Circumcision in the Female: It's a Necessity and How to Perform it." *American Journal of Clinical Medicine,* vol. 22, no. 6, pp. 520-523, June 1915.

Prakash S, [sic: Parkash], Jeyakumar S, Subraman K, Chauldhuri S, "Human subpreputal collection: its and function." 110, *J Urol*, 211-212, (1973).

Wayne, Eileen, "Understanding Urinary Tract Infections," *Infect Urology*, 8 (4), 111, 114-120, 1995.

West DC, "Cliteroidectomy," *BMJ*, 2: 585, 1866.

White C, "Little evidence for effectiveness of scientific peer review," *BMJ*, 2003: 326-341 (1 February).

PSYCHOLOGY

Alhassan, Amina, "The plague called transfer of aggression," *Daily Trust*, Oct 2, 2010.

American Psychiatric Association, "Shared Psychotic Disorder," American Psychiatric Association Diagnostic and Statistical Manual of Mental Disorders, Fifth Edition *DSM 5*, Arlington, p. 122.

American Psychiatric Association, "Delusional Disorder," *American P sychiatric Association. Diagnostic and Statistical Manual of Mental Diso rders, Fifth Edition (DSM-5)*, American Psychiatric Association, Arlingt on, 2013.

Beauman, Jennifer, "Psychological Projection: Dealing with Undesirable Emotions," *Everyday Health*, November 15, 2017.

Canserver G, "Psychological effects of circumcision," 38, *Brit J Med Psych*, 321-331, (1965).

Daly, "The Psycho-biological Origins of Circumcision," 31, *International J Psychoanalysis*, 217, (1950).

deMause, Lloyd, "Childhood and Cultural Evolution," *The Journal of Psychohistory*, Vol. 26, No. 3, Winter 1999.

deMause, Lloyd, *The Social Altar*, Presented at the 18th Annual Convention of the International Psychohistorical Association, June 7, 1995, New York City.

deMause, Lloyd, "The Universality of Incest," Th*e Journal of Psychohistory*, Fall 1991, Vol. 19, No. 2, 123-144.

deMause, Lloyd, "Why Cults Terrorize and Kill Children," *The Journal of Psychohistory*, 21 (4) 1994.

Diekmann, Andreas and Przepiorka, Wojtek, "Punitive preferences, monetary incentives and tacit coordination in the punishment of defectors promote coordination in humans," *PubMed*, US gov., 19 May 2015.

Dolan, Eric W., "Collective narcissism can warp your moral judgments, according to new psychology research," *Social Psychology*, PsyPost, July 8, 2021.

Flaherty J, "Circumcision and Schizophrenia," *J Clin Psychiatry*, 1980, 41: 96-98.

Goldman R, "The psychological impact of circumcision," 83, Supplement, 1, *BJU International*, 92-102, (1999).

Gunnar MR, Frisch RO, Korsvik S, Donhowe JM, "The effects of circumcision on serum cortical and behavior," *Psychoneuroendocrinology*, 1981, 6: 269-75.

Lund, C.A., Gardiner, A.G., (1977). "The Gaslight Phenomenon: An Institutional Variant." *British Journal of Psychiatry*, 131 (5): 533-34.

Monaghan, Conal; Bizumic, Boris; Selborn, Martin (2016). "The role of Machiavellian views and tactics in psychopathy". *Personality and Individual Differences*, 94: 72-81.

Newman, Leonard S., Duff, Kimberley J., Baumeister, Roy F., (1997). "A new look at defensive projection: Thought suppression, accessibility, and biased person perception". *Journal of Personality and Social Psychology*, 72(5): 980-1001.

Ray, John J., "Punitive Personality Disorder," *The Journal of Social Psychology*, 1985, 125(3), 329-333.

Roberts, Craig; Vakirtzis, Antonios; Kristjansdottir, Havlicek, Jan, "Who Punishes? Personality traits predict individual variation in punitive sentiment," *Evol. Psychology*, 2013 Feb 18,11(1): 168-200.

Summit, R. C., "The child sexual abuse accommodation syndrome," *Child Abuse Neglect*, 1983:7(2):177-93.

Talbert J, et al., "Adrenal cortical response to circumcision in the neonate," *Obstet Gynecol*, 48: 208-10, Aug 1976.

Vanderbilt, D.; Augustyn, M., "The Effects of Bullying," *Paediatrics and Child Health*, 20 (7): 315-320, 2010.

Vankin, Shmeul (Sam), *Malignant Self-Love: Narcissism Revisited*, Narcissist Publications, 2007.

Williams, Ray (3 May 2011). "The Silent Epidemic: Workplace Bullying," *Psychology Today*.

SOCIAL - PARENTAL

Belsky, J, "Child maltreatment: An ecological integration," *American Psychologist*, 35(4), 320-335.

Bocian, Konrad; Cichocka, Alexandra; Wojciszke, Bogdan, "Moral Tribalism: Moral judgments of actions supporting ingroup interests depend on collectivism", *Journal of Experimental Social Psychology*, V. 93, March 2021.

Bolande RP, "Ritualistic Surgery: Circumcision and Tonsilectomy," *New England Journal of Medicine,* 1969: 280: 591-596.

Boykoff, Jules, *Suppression of Descent: How the State and Mass Media Squelch US American Social Movements*, New Approaches in Sociology, Routledge, 2006.

Brown J, "A Cross-cultural study of female initiation rites," *Am Anthropol*, 65, 837-53, 1963.

deMause L, "The History of Child Abuse," *The Journal of Psychohistory*, 25 (3), Winter, 1998.

Gollaher DL, "From Ritual to Science: The Medical Transformation of Circumcision in America," *Journal of Social History*, Vol. 28, No., 1, pp. 5-36, Fall, 1994.

Loeb L, "The Blood Sacrifice Complex, Memoirs," *Am Anthropological Assoc*, #30, 1923.

Montague A, "Ritual Mutilation Among Primitive Peoples," *Cibia Symposium*, October 1946, pp. 421-436.x

Paige K, "The Ritual of Circumcision," *Human Nature*, May, 1978: 40.

Slater, Philip E, "On Social Regression," *Am Socio Review*, 28, June 1963, p.249.

Tobin, Theresa Weynand, "Cultural Imperialism," *Encyclopedia Britannica*, within, The Editors of Encyclopaedia. "Social mobility". *Encyclopedia Britannica*, 22 May. 2020.

Rothenberg MB, "Is there an Unconscious National Conspiracy Against Children in the United States," *Clin Peditatr*, 1980: 19: 10-24.

170

Slater, Philip E, "On Social Regression," *Am Socio Review*, 28, June 1963, p. 13.

Thomas WI, "Sex in Primitive Morality," *American Journal of Sociology*, 4, (1899): 774-787.

Thomas WI, "The Relation of Sex to Primitive Social Control," *American Journal of Sociology*, 3, (1898): 754-76.

Thomas WI, "The Relation of the Medicine Man to the Origin of the Professional Occupations," *Decennial Publications of the University of Chicago*, First Series, 4 (1903): 241-256.

Wood DP, "Sexual Abuse during Childhood and Adolescence and its effects on the Physical and Emotional Quality of Life of the Survivor: A Review o0f the Literature," *Military Medicine*, Vol. 161, October 1996, pp. 582-587.

Wallerstein E, "Is Non Religious circumcision necessary?," *J Am Acad Child Psychiatry*, 1985, 24: (3): 264-5.

SURGICAL COMPLICATIONS

Adams J, et al., "Fournier's gangrene in children," *Urology*, 35:439, 1990.

Anday E, Kobori J, "Staphylococcal scalded skin syndrome: a complication of circumcision," *Clinical Pediatrics*, Phila., 1982, 21: 420.

Amon R, et al., "Unilateral leg cyanosis: an unusual complication of circumcision," *Eur J Pediatr*, 1992: 151-716.

Attalla M, Taweela M, "Pathogenesis of post-circumcision adhesion," *Pediatr Surg Int*, 1994, 9, 103-105.

Berman W, "Urinary retention due to ritual circumcision," (Letter), *Pediatrics*, October 1975, 56: 621.

Bliss D, Healey J, Waldhausen J, "Necrotizing fasciitis after Plastibell circumcision." *J Pediatrics*, 1997, 131, 459-462.

Braun D, "Neonatal bacteremia and circumcision, *Pediatrics*, 1990, 85: 135-6.

Cleary DG, Kold S, "Overwhelming infection with group B beta-hemolytic strepoccus associated with circumcision," *Pediatrics*, Vol. 64, no. 3, Sept. 1970: 301-302.

Cleary TG, Kold S, "Circumcision Disasters," *Pediatrics*, 1980 65: 1053-4.

Craig J, et al., "Acute obstructive uropathy – a rare complication of circumcision," *Eur J Pediatrics*, 1994, 153: 360-71.

Editor, "Hazards of circumcisions," *Practitioner*, 1967: 198:611.

Eldin, Usama Saad, "Post-circumcision keloid – A Case Report," *Annals of Burns and Fire Disasters*, vol. XII, no. 3, September 1999.

Gold S, "Bleeding after circumcision," *Canadian Medical Journal*, 1940: 43: 473.

Goldman M, et al., "Urinary tract infection following ritual Jewish circumcision," *Israel J of Med Sci*, 1996, 32(11): 1098-1102.

Gosden M, "Tetanus following circumcision," *Trans R Soc Trop Med Hyg*, 1935, 28: 645-8.

Kirkpatrick BV, Eitamin DV, "Neonatal Septicemia After Circumcision," *Clinical Pediatrics*, 13: 767, 1974.

Lewis EL, "Tuberculosis of the penis: a report of 5 new cases, and a complete review of the literature," *J of Urology*, 1946: 56: 737-745.

Marsh SK, Archer TJ, "Bipolar diathermy haemostasis during circumcision," *British J of Surgery*, 1995: 82: 533.

172

Michelowski R., "Silica granuloma at the site of circumcision for phimosis: a case report," *Dermatologica*, 1983, 166: 261-3.

Mor A, et al., "Tachycardia and heart failure after circumcision," *Arch Dis Child*, 1987, 62: 80-81,

Ngan J, Waldhausen J, Santucci, "I think this child has an infected penis after neonatal circumcision," *Online Pediatric Urology*, April 1996.

Ozbek N, Sarikayalar, F, "Toxic methaemoglobinaemia after circumcision," *European J of Pediatrics*, 1993, 152: 80.

Ozdemir E, "Significant increased complication risk with mass circumcision," *BJU*, vol. 80, 136-139, August 1997.

Pearlman C, "Caution advised in electrocautery circumcision," *Urology*, 1982, 19: 453.

Pinkham E, Stevenson A, "Unusual reaction to local anesthesia: gangrene of the prepuce," *US Armed Forces Med J*, 1958, 9: 120-2.

Ponsky J, Ross J, Knipper N, et al., "A Natural History of Penile Adhesions after Circumcision," (Presentation: *1999 Amer Urol Assoc*).

Reuben M, "Tuberculosis Following Ritual Circumcision," *Arch Pediatr*, 34: 186, 1917.

Rosenstein H, "Wound Diphtheria in the Newborn Infant Following Circumcision," *J Pediatrics*, 18: 657, 1948.

Ruff M, et al., "Myocardial injury following immediate postnatal circumcision," *Am J Obstet & Gynecol*, 1982, 144: 850-1.

Sauer LW, "Fatal Staphylococcous Bronchopneumonia Following Ritual Circumcision," *Am J Ob & Gyn*, 46: 583, 1943.

Scurlock JM, Pemberton PJ, "Neonatal Meningitis and Circumcision," *Medical Journal of Australia*, (1977): 332-334.

Sharpe JR, Finnet RP, "Electrocautery Circumcision," *Urology*, 19 (1982): 228.

Smith GI, Greenup R, Takafuji ET, "Circumcision As A Risk Factor for Urethritis in Racial Groups," *American Journal of Public Health*, 77: 452-454, 1987.

Snellman I, Stang H, "Prospective evaluation of complications of dorsal penile nerve block for neonatal circumcision," *Pediatrics*, 1995, 95: 705-8.

Stranko J, et al., "Impetigo in newborn infants associated with a plastic bell clamp circumcision," *Pediatr Infect Dis*, 1986, 5: 597-9.

Sussman SJ, Schiller RP, Shashikumaro VI, "Fournier's syndrome: Report of three cases and review of the literature," 132, *Am J Dis Child*, 1189-1191, (1978).

Taylor PK, "Herpes Genitalis and circumcision," *British J Venereal Dis*, 51: 274-277, 1975.

Trier W, Drach G, "Concealed Penis: Another Complication of Circumcision," *Amer J Dis Child*, 125: 276, 1973.

Van Howe RS, "Is circumcision Healthy - No," *Priorities*, vol. 9, no. 4, 1997.

Walfisch, et al., "Complications of ritual circumcision," *BJU*, 77, June 1996, 924.

Warwick DJ, Dickson WA, "Keloid of the penis after circumcision," *Postgraduate Medical Journal*, 1993: 69: 236-7.

William K, Kapila I, "Complications of Circumcision," *British Journal of Surgery*, vol. 80, pp. 1231-1236, Oct. 1993.xx

Wiswell T, et al., "Staphylococcus aureus after neonatal circumcision in relation to device used," *J Pediatr*, 1991, 119: 302-4.

Woodside J, "Circumcision Disasters." *Pediatrics*, (Springfield Illinois), vol. 64, no. 5, May 1980, 1053-4.

Woodside J, "Necrotizing fasciitis after neonatal circumcision," *Am J Dis Child*, 134-301, 1980.

Endnotes

FIRST DO NO HARM

[1] *Stedman's Medical Dictionary*, 21st Edition, Williams & Wilkins, Baltimore, MD, 1966, p. 738.

INTRODUCTION

[2] Glick, Leonard, *Marked in Your Flesh: Circumcision from Ancient Judea to Modern America*, Oxford University Press2005.

[3] Edinger, Edward, Ego and Archetype, *Shambala*, 1992, pp. 3-4.

[4] Renfrew, C., & Bahn, P., *Archaeology: Theories, Methods, and Practice*, Thames & Hudson, 2016.

[5] Klass, D, & Goss, R., *Dead but not lost: Grief narratives in religious traditions*, AltaMira Press, 1999.

[6] Watson, JL, Rawski, ES, *Death Ritual in Late Imperial and Modern China*. University of California Press, 1988.

[7] Mbiti, J, *African Religions & Philosophy*. Heinemann, 1990.

[8] Jung, CG, *Symbols of Transformation*, Princeton University Press, Bollingen Series XX, 1990, pp. 235 and 431.

ISLAM

[9] "Shared Psychotic Disorder," *American Psychiatric Association Diagnostic and Statistical Manual of Mental Disorders*, Fifth Edition *DSM 5*, Arlington, p. 122.

[10] "Delusional Disorder," *American Psychiatric Association. Diagnostic and Statistical Manual of Mental Disorders*, Fifth Edition (*DSM-5*), American Psychiatric Association, Arlington 2013.

[11] Estes, Clarissa Pinkola (Studies in Jungian Psychology), *Women Who Run With the Wolves: Myths and Stories of the Wild Woman Archetype*, Ballentine, 1995.

[12] Weiser, Kathy, "The Ghost Dance – A Promise of Fulfillment," *Legends of America*, February 2020.

[13] Young, Gloria A., *The Encyclopedia of Oklahoma History and Culture*, "Ghost Dance," Oklahoma Historical Society.

[14] Duignan, Brian, Editor, *Encyclopedia Britannica*, "Ghost Dance: North American Indian cult."

[15] Tikkanen, Amy, *Encyclopedia Britannica*, "Sun Dance: religious ceremony."

[16] Campbell, Joseph, *The Power of Myth*, Doubleday, 1988. Original video available.

[17] Quanta, Ahmed, "And Now: Female Genital Mutilation Comes to America," *Daily Beast*, May 5, 2017.

[18] Shell-Duncan, Bettina, "The medicalization of female "circumcision": harm reduction or promotion of a dangerous practice," *Social Science & Medicine*, Volume 52, Issue 7, April 2001, Pages 1013-1028.

[19] Serourx, G. I., "Medicalization of female genital mutilation/cutting," *African Journal of Urology*, Volume 19, Issue 3, September 2013, Pages 145-149.

[20] Brownies, Sharon, "In the Name of Ritual: An Unprecedented Legal Case focuses on Genital Politics," *U.S. News and World Report*.

[21] Bocian, Konrad; Cichocka, Alexandra; Wojciszke, Bogdan, "Moral Tribalism: Moral judgments of actions supporting ingroup interests depend on collectivism", *Journal of Experimental Social Psychology*, Volume 93, March 2021.

[22] Beauman, Jennifer, "Psychological Projection: Dealing with Undesirable Emotions," *Everyday Health*, November 15, 2017.

[23] Newman, Leonard S., Duff, Kimberley J., Baumeister, Roy F., (1997). "A new look at defensive projection: Thought suppression, accessibility, and biased person perception". *Journal of Personality and Social Psychology*, 72(5): 980-1001.

[24] U.S. Department of Justice, "Dignity Health Agrees to Pay $37 Million to Settle False Claims Act Allegations", *Office of Public Affairs*, Oct. 30, 2014.

[25] Bertaux-Navoiseau, Michel Herve, **The Koran forbids excision and circumcision:** (français): Le Coran contre les mutilations sexuelles (mis à jour 06.01.2023) |. *Academia.edu*.

[26] Sternberg, Robert J, "Ethical Drift," *Association of American Colleges & Universities,* Summer 2012, Vol. 98, No. 3.

[27] Kleinman, Carole, "Ethical Drift: When Good People Do Bad Things," *JONA's Healthcare Law, Ethics, and Regulation.* 8(3):72-76, Jully 2006.

[28] Beasley, Brett, "Keep ethics from "fading" when you face a tough decision," *University of Notre Dame*, Notre Dame Deloitte for Ethical Leadership, Mendoza College of Business, 2023.

[29] Detert JR, Trevin LK, Sweitzer VL, "Moral Disengagement in Ethical Decision Making: A Study of Antecedents and Outcomes," *Journal of Applied Psychology*, Vol. 93, No. 2 pp. 374-391.

[30] Babazadeh, Natasha, "Concealing Evidence: 'Parallel Construction,' Federal Investigations, and the Constitution," *Virginia Journal of Law &Technology*, University of Virginia, Fall 2018, Vol.22, No. 01

[31] Beauman, Jennifer, "Psychological Projection: Dealing with Undesirable Emotions," *Everyday Health*, November 15, 2017.

[32] Newman, Leonard S., Duff, Kimberley J., Baumeister, Roy F., (1997). "A new look at defensive projection: Thought suppression, accessibility, and biased person perception". *Journal of Personality and Social Psychology*, 72(5): 980-1001.

[33] Monaghan, Conal; Bizumic, Boris; Selborn, Martin (2016). "The role of Machiavellian views and tactics in psychopathy". *Personality and Individual Differences*, 94: 72-81.

[34] Lund, C.A., Gardiner, A.G., (1977). "The Gaslight Phenomenon: An Institutional Variant." *British Journal of Psychiatry*, 131 (5): 533-34.

[35] Stern, Robin, (2007). "The Gaslight Effect: How to Spot and Survive the Hidden Manipulation Others Use to Control Your Life," *Random House*.

[36] Dorpat, Theodore L. (1996). *Gaslighting, the Double Whammy, Interrogation, and Other Methods of Covert Control in Psychotherapy and Psychoanalysis*, Jason Aronson, 1996.

[37] Maren S (2001). "Neurobiology of Pavlovian fear conditioning". *Annual Review of Neuroscience*. **24**: 897–931.

[38] Wallace KJ, Rosen JB (October 2000). "Predator odor as an unconditioned fear stimulus in rats: elicitation of freezing by trimethylthiazoline, a component of fox feces". *Behavioral Neuroscience*. **114** (5): 912–22.

[39] Williams, Ray (3 May 2011). "The Silent Epidemic: Workplace Bullying," *Psychology Today*.

[40] Stale, Einarsen (2003). *Bullying and Emotional Abuse in the Workplace: International Perspectives in Research and Practice*, Taylor & Francis.

[41] Vanderbilt, D.; Augustyn, M., "The Effects of Bullying," *Paediatrics and Child Health*, 20 (7): 315-320, 2010.

[42] Summit, R. C., "The child sexual abuse accommodation syndrome," Child Abuse Negl., 1983:7(2):177-93.

[43] Alhassan, Amina, "The plague called transfer of aggression," *Daily Trust*, Oct 2 2010.

[44] Tobin, Theresa Weynand, "Cultural Imperialism," *Encyclopedia Britannica*, within, The Editors of Encyclopaedia. "Social mobility". *Encyclopedia Britannica*, 22 May. 2020.

[45] Eliade, Mircea, *The Myth of the Eternal Return*, Princeton University Press, Bollingen Series XLVI, 1954, pp. 32 and 76.

[46] Schwartz, W., *Pediatric Primary Care: A Problem-Solving Approach*, 2nd edition, Year Book Medical Publishers, Chicago, IL, 1990, p. 861.

[47] Lifton, Robert Jay, *The Nazi Doctors: Medical Killing and the Psychology of Genocide*, Basic Books, New York, NY, 1986, pp. 418, 422, 423, and 488.

[48] Ausubel, Kenny, *When Healing Becomes a Crime*, Healing Arts Press, 2000, p. 291.

[49] deMause, Lloyd, *The Emotional Life of Nations*, Chapter 7, (Part 2: "Childhood and Cultural Evolution," Originally in: *The Journal of Psychohistory*, v. 26, N. 3, Winter 1999.)

[50] Bittles AH, *A Background Summary on Cosanguineous Marriage*, Center for Human
Genetics, Edith Cowan, University of Perth, Australia WA 6027, May, 2001.

[51] Swinford, Steven, "First cousin marriages in Pakiatani communities to 'appalling' disabilities among children," *Telegraph*, 07 July 2015.

[52] Pellissier, Hank, "Cousin Marriage – 70% in Pakistan – Should it be Prohibited?," *Institute for Ethics and Emerging Technologies*, 26 May 2012.

[53] Dolan, Eric W., "Collective narcissism can warp your moral judgments, according to new psychology research," *Social Psychology*, PsyPost, July 8, 2021.

[54] Goodman, Richard Merle, *Genetic Disorders among the Jewish People*, The Johns Hopkins University Press, 1979.

[55] Abel, Ernest L. *Jewish Genetic Disorders: A Layman's Guide*, Published by McFarland & Company, Jefferson, NC (2008)

[56] Barnard GW and Kripel JJ, editors, *Crossing Boundaries: Essays on the Ethical Status of Mysticism*, Chatham House, London, UK, 2002.

[57] Monteleone, James A., *Recognition of Child Abuse for the Mandated Reporter*, Second Edition, G. W. Medical Publishing, Inc., 1996, p. 157.

[58] Forward, Susan with Buck, Craig, *Toxic Parents: Overcoming Their Hurtful Legacy and Reclaiming Your Life*, Bantam, New York, NY, pp. 15-17, 19, 5-6, 11, 5, 130 and 6.

[59] Bittles AH, A *Background Summary on Cosanguineous Marriage, Centre for Human Genetics*, Edith Cowan, University Perth Australia WA 6027, May, 2001.

[60] Adams, Kenneth, *Silently Seduced: When Parents Make Their Children Partners: Understanding Covert Incest*, HCI, Deerfield Beach, FL, 1991.

[61] Miller, RK, *Collection of Tears*, Nunzio Press, Eugene, OR, 2006.

[62] deMause, Lloyd, "The Universality of Incest," *The Journal of Psychohistory*, Fall, 1991, vol. 19, No. 2. Included is a reference to: Landes, David S, "The Wealth and Poverty of Nations: Why Some are Rich and Some are Poor," pp. 6-14.

[63] Williams, John Alden, *The Word of Islam*, University of Texas Press. Austin. TX, 1994.

[64] Farah, Caesar e., *Islam*, Barrons Educational Series, Great Neck, NY, 1994.

[65] Kitahara, Michio, "A Cross-Cultural Test of the Freudian Theory of Circumcision," *International Journal of Psychoanalytic Psychotherapy,* 5(1976):535-46.

[66] deMause, Lloyd, The History of Child Abuse, The Journal of Psychohistory, 25 (Winter) 1998.

[67] Burney, Robert, *Codependence: The Dance of Wounded Souls*, Joy to You &Me Enterprises, Cambria, CA, 1995.

[68] Love, Patricia, Jo, *The Emotional Incest Syndrome*, Bantam, New York, NY, 1991, p. 126.

[69] deMause, Lloyd, "The Universality of Incest."

[70] deMause, Lloyd, *Foundation of Psychohistory*, Creative Roots, 1982.

[71] Eliade, Mircea, *The Myth of the Eternal Return*, Princeton University Press, Princeton, NJ, 1954.

[72] deMause, Lloyd, "Why Cults Terrorize and Kill Children," *The Journal of Psychohistory*, 21 (4) 1994.

[73] deMause, Lloyd, *The Social Altar*, Presented at the 18th Annual Convention of the International Psychohistorical Association, 7 June 1995 in New York City.

[74] Kitahara, Michio, "A Cross-Cultural Test of the Freudian Theory of Circumcision,"
International Journal of Psychoanalytic Psychotherapy, 5(1976): 535-546.

[75] Neumann, Erich, *The Great Mother*, Princeton University Press, Bollingen Series XLVII, 1991, p.72.

RITUAL

[76] Campbell, Joseph, *Primitive Mythology: The Masks of God*, Penguin Arkana, NY, NY, 1959, PP. 283-297 and 319-322.

[77] Bell, Catherine, *Ritual Theory, Ritual Practice*, Oxford University Press, 1992, p. 215.

[78] Ibid, pp. 215, 102, and 197.

[79] Ibid, Bell referencing Pierre *Bourdieu's Outline of a Theory of Practice*, Cambridge University Press, Cambridge, UK, 1977, pp. 120, 207 (and Note 75), and 111.

[80] Ibid, pp. 173-174.

[81] Dr. Joyce Brothers, *Today*, 28 October 1996.

[82] Bell, Catherine, Ritual Theory, *Ritual Practice*, p. 106.

[83] Ibid, Bell referencing Steven Lukes "Political Rituals and Social Integration," *Journal of the British Sociological Association*, 9, no. 2, (1975), pp. 289-29-, 300, and 305.

[84] Ibid, p. 96.

ACCULTURATION

[85] Campbell, Joseph, *The Power of Myth*, Doubleday, New York, NY, 1988, p. 48.

[86] Van der Kolk B, "The Compulsion to Repeat the Trauma: Re-enactment, Revctimization, and Masochism." Psychiatric Clinics of North America, Volume 12, Number 2, Pages 389-411, June 1989.

[87] Goldman R, "The psychological impact of circumcision," *BJU International*, Volume 83, Supplement 1, Pages 93-102, January 1, 1999.

[88] Menage, Janet, "Circumcision and Psychological Harm," NOR*M-UK*.

[89] Jacobson B, Eklund G, Hamburger L, Linnarsson D, Sedvall G, Valverius M, "Perinatal origin of adult self-destructive behavior," *Acta Psychiatr Scand*, Vol. 76, No, 42, pp. 364-371, October 1987.

[90] Neppe VM, Smith ME, "Culture, Psychopathology and Psi: A Clinical Relational Relationship," *Parapsychological J of S.A,,* 1982, 3:1, 1-5, edited.

[91] Fongay, Peter, "The transgenerational transmission of holocaust trauma," *Attachment &Human Development*, Vol. 1, No. 1, April 1999, pp. 92-114(23).

[92] Crawford, Christina and Bradshaw, John, *No Safe Place: The Legacy of Family Violence*, Barrytown/Station Hill Press, 1994.

[93] Mishra, Vinod, *Is Male Circumcision Protective of HIV?*, Presented at the 16th International AIDS Conference (AIDS) 2006, Toronto, Canada.

[94] Ray, John J., "The Punitive Personality," J. Social Psych, 125(3), 329-333.

[95] Schwartz W., Charney E, et al., *Pediatric Primary Care: A Problem-solving Approach, Year Book*, Medical Publishers, 1990, Chicago, pp. 861-862.

[96] Jung, Carl G., The Undiscovered Self, Mentor, 1958, pp. 16-17.

[97] Lukes, Steven, "Political Rituals and Social Integration," *Journal of the British Sociological Association*, 9, no. 2, (1975), pp. 289-291, 300 and 305.

[98] Landau, Elaine, *Child Abuse: An American Epidemic*, J Messner, 1990.

[99] Eliade, Mircea, *The Myth of the Eternal Return*, Princeton University Press, Bollingen Series XLVI, 1954, pp. 32 and 76.

[100] Honko, Lauri, "The problem of defining myth," *Scripta Instituti Donneriani Aboensis*, 6 January 1972

[101] Losada, José Manuel and Lipscomb, Antonella, *Myth and Emotions*, Cambridge Scholars Publishing, 2017.

[102] Hollis, James, Under Saturn's Shadow: The Wounding and Healing of Men, (Studies in Jungian Psychology by Jungian Analysts), Inner City Books, 1994.

[103] Edinger, Edward, *The Mystery of THE CONIUNCTIO Alchemical Image of Individuation*, Inner City Books, 1922.

[104] Ray, John J., "Punitive Personality Disorder," *The Journal of Social Psychology*, 1985, 125 (3), 329-333.

JUDAISM

[105] Bell, Catherine, *Ritual Theory, Ritual Practice*, Oxford University Press, 1992, pp. 23 and 26.

[106] Neumann, Erich, *The Great Mother*, Princeton University Press, *1991*.

MUNCHAUSEN COMPLEX

[107] Asher, Richard (1951), "Munchausen Syndrome," *The Lancet*, i: 339-41.

[108] American Psychiatric Association, *Quick Reference to the: Diagnostic Criteria From DSM-IV*, American Psychiatric Publishing, Washington, DC, 1994, p. 227.

[109] Meadow, Roy, (1977), "Munchausen Syndrome by Proxy: The Hinterland of Child Abuse," *The Lancet*, ii: 342-5.

[110] American Psychiatric Association, *Quick Reference to the: Diagnostic Criteria From DSM-IV*, American Psychiatric Publishing, Washington, DC, 1994, p. 228.

[111] Libow JA, Schreier HA, (1986), "Three Forms of Factitious Illness in Children: When is it Munchausen Syndrome by Proxy?," *American Journal of Orthopsychiatry*, 56(4):602:11.

[112] Douglas, John with Olshaker, Mark, *Journey into Darkness*, Pocket Books, NY, p. 75.

[113] Tantum D, Whittaker J, "Personality Disorder and Self-wounding," *British Journal of Psychiatry*, 1992, 161,451-464.

[114] deMause, Lloyd, "The Universality of Incest," *The Journal of Psychohistory,* Fall 1991, Vol. 19, No. 2.

CRIMINOLOGY

[115] Monteleone, James A., *Recognition of Child Abuse for the Mandated Reporter*, G.W. Medical Publishing, Inc., St. Louis, MO, 1996, p.1.

[116] Dawkins, Richard, *The Selfish Gene*, Oxford University Press, Oxford, 1976.

[117] Evans, Colin, *The Casebook of Forensic Detection: Hoe Science Solved 100 of the World's Most Baffling Crimes*, John Wiley & Sons, NY, 1996, p. 17.

[118] Reid WH, "Myths About Violent Sexual Predators and All That Pesky Legislation," *J Pract Psychiatry and Behav Health*, July 1998, 4:246-248.

CRIMINOLOGY

[119] Monteleone, James A., *Recognition of Child Abuse for the Mandated Reporter*, G.W. Medical Publishing, Inc., St. Louis, MO, 1996, p. 1.

[120] Douglas, John with Olshaker, Mark, *Obsession*, pp. 33-34.

[121] Fletcher, Connie, *What Cops Know*, Pocket, NY, 1996, pp. 118 and 130.

[122] Frazer, James George, *The Belief in Immortality and the Worship of the Dead*, Macmillan, New York, NY, p. 254.

[123] Graves, Robert, *The Greek Myths*, Complete Edition, Penguin, New York, NY, 1992, p. 119.

[124] Douglas, John with Olshaker, Mark, *The Anatomy of Motive*, Pocket Books, New York, NY, 1999, pp. 279, 262, 289-313, and 367.

[125] Douglas, John with Olshaker, Mark, *Obsession*, pp. 332-333.

[340] Vakin, Shmuel (Sam), *Malignant Self Love: Narcissism Revisited*, Narcissist Pub., Czech Republic, 2003.

[127] Douglas, John with Olshaker, Mark, *Journey into Darkness*, Pocket, NY, 1995, pp. 33-34, 43, 66 and 75.

[128] Douglas, John with Olshaker, Mark, *Obsession*, p. 13.

[129] Bell, Catherine, *Ritual Theory, Ritual Practice*, Oxford University Press, Oxford University Press, Oxford, UK, 1992.

MEDICAL

[130] Bell, Catherine, Ritual Theory, Ritual Practice, Oxford University Press, 1992. Bell referenced: Bordieu, Pierre's book: *Outline of a Theory of Practice*, Cambridge University Press, Cambridge, UK, 1977, pp. 184, 40-41, 207, 98-108.

LEGAL

[131] Schroeder, Patricia & Collins, Barbara, *The Federal Prohibition of Female Circumcision Mutilation Act of 113, (HR 3247)*.

[132] Spath, HJ, Smith, EC, HarperCollins College Outline: *The Constitution of the United States*, 13th edition, p. 211, Amendment IX, (1868), Section 1, HarperCollins, New York, NY, 1991.

[133] Kay, Susan, *The Constitutional Dimensions of an Inmate's Rights to Health Care*, National Commission on Correctional Health Care, 1991, p. 5.

[134] Gifis, Steven H, *Law Dictionary*, 2nd edition, Barron's Educational Series, Hauppauge, NY, 1984, p. 16.

[135] Harrison, James, "Benefit for burn victim scheduled," *The Ukiah Daily Journal*, Ukiah, CA, 16 October 2001.

[136] Thevenot, Carri Geer, "Father fights to stop son's circumcision," Las Vegas Review-Journal, Las Vegas, NV, 15 January 2001.

[137] Gifis, Steven H, *Law Dictionary*, 2nd edition, Barron's Educational Series, Hauppauge, NY, 1984, p. 240.

[138] Gifis, SH, p. 62-63.

[139] Gifis SH, p. 76.

[140] White, Becky Cox, *Competence to Consent*, Georgetown University Press, Washington, DC, 1994, pp. 16,27-28, 49 and 154.

[141] Pozgar, George D., *Legal Aspects of Health Care Administration*, Aspen, Rockville, MD, 1990, pp. 336. 264-66.

[142] Svoboda, Steven, "*Doctor pays parents $23,000 for circumcision without consent*," NOCIRC press release, (15 September 2006).

[143] Gifis, SH, p. 172.

[144] Gifis, SH, p.194-195.

[145] *Hate Crime: The Violence of Intolerance*, (15 September 2006) Department of Justice.

[146] Gifis, SH, p. 240.

[147] Gifis, SH, p. 288.

[148] Zimmerman, F., "Origin and Significance of the Jewish Rite of Circumcision," *Psychoanalytic Review*, 38(2): 103-112, 1951.

[149] Douglas J, Ressler, RK, et al., *Sexual Homicide: Patterns and Motives*, Jossey-Bass, San Francisco, CA, 1992, p. 48.

[150] Gifis, SH, p. 289.

[151] Cronin, Danielle, "Circumcision victim's bid to help others," *The Canberra Times*, Canberra, Australia, 31 March 2002.

[152] Gifis SH, p. 309-310.